MANAGING CHRONIC PAIN

Strategies for Dealing with

- **Back Pain** ■ **Headaches**
- **Muscle & Joint Pain**
- **Cancer Pain**
- **Abdominal Pain**

Siang-Yang Tan, Ph.D.

InterVarsity Press
Downers Grove, Illinois

4/98 Gen Fund $10.00

InterVarsity Press® is the book-publishing division of InterVarsity Christian Fellowship®, a student movement active on campus at hundreds of universities, colleges and schools of nursing in the United States of America, and a member movement of the International Fellowship of Evangelical Students. For information about local and regional activities, write Public Relations Dept., InterVarsity Christian Fellowship, 6400 Schroeder Rd., P.O. Box 7895, Madison, WI 53707-7895.

ISBN 0-8308-1989-4

Printed in the United States of America ⊗

Library of Congress Cataloging-in-Publication Data

Tan, Siang-Yang, 1954-
   Managing chronic pain/Siang-Yang Tan.
      p.   cm.
   Includes bibliographical references.
   ISBN 0-8308-1989-4 (pbk.: alk. paper)
   1. Chronic pain.
   RB127.T365   1996
   616'.0472—dc20   96-22370
                                              CIP

18	17	16	15	14	13	12	11	10	9	8	7	6	5	4	3	2	1
11	10	09	08	07	06	05	04	03	02	01	00	99	98	97	96		

To my mother, Madam Chiow Yang Quek,
who has suffered various pains in her life,
with my deepest appreciation and love,
and to the memory of my late father, Siew Thiam Tan.

To my siblings: Sien Chuan Tan and his family;
Siang Chik Tan and his family; Siang Yong Tan and his family;
Daisy Ng and her family; Gek Huan Tan;
and to the memory of my late sister Gek Hong Tan,
who endured much suffering and pain during her lifetime.

And to my uncle and his wife, Mr. and Mrs. Kee Tan,
and their daughter, Gek Yeong Tan.

I deeply appreciate all of you and thank God for you!

Acknowledgments

I would like to acknowledge with deep gratitude the help of Kim Roth, my former secretary at the Graduate School of Psychology, Fuller Theological Seminary, who faithfully deciphered my handwritten scribbles and transformed them into clearly legible words through her skillful use of the word processor/computer. Linda Rojas, my present secretary, typed the final drafts of the book. The editorial assistance and support of Andy Le Peau and Linda Doll at InterVarsity Press, as well as helpful feedback from three anonymous reviewers of an earlier draft of the book, are also gratefully acknowledged.

The significant and tremendous contributions of Dr. Ronald Melzack to pain research and treatment cannot be overemphasized. I was blessed to have him as one of my mentors and dissertation supervisors (together with Dr. Ernest G. Poser) while I was a graduate student in the Ph.D. program in clinical psychology at McGill University (1976-1980). His influence on me and my own work in the area of pain, especially as reflected in the writing of this book, is deeply appreciated. I would also like to acknowledge the invaluable contributions that Dr. Ernest G. Poser made to my scholarly and professional development as a clinical psychologist and to my training in cognitive-behavior therapy.

Finally, I want to express my sincere thanks to my wife, Angela, and my children, Carolyn and Andrew, for their faithful support, patience, love and prayers as I continue to write. And most of all, my greatest thanksgiving to Jesus Christ, my Lord and Savior, for helping me to finish writing this book on pain. He alone ultimately is the answer to the challenge of pain and all our other struggles.

Preface

I have written this book on managing chronic pain from a Christian perspective, primarily for people suffering from various chronic-pain conditions. I trust and pray that it will be a real help and blessing to them.

My doctoral dissertation, completed in 1980 at McGill University in Montreal, Quebec, Canada, was on the topic of cognitive-behavioral skills training for acute pain (see Siang-Yang Tan and Ernest G. Poser, "Acute Pain in a Clinical Setting: Effects of Cognitive-Behavioural Skills Training," *Behaviour Research and Therapy* 20 (1982): 535-45). Dr. Ernest G. Poser and Dr. Ronald Melzack were my dissertation advisors.

It has been a good experience to pull together my earlier training in pain treatment and cognitive-behavior therapy with more recent research and advances in pain management, and to integrate all of these within a biblical framework of God's power and healing, as well as God's grace and suffering, in the ongoing challenge of pain. My hope and prayer are that many Christians as well as others suffering from various chronic-pain conditions will find deep comfort and practical help through this book. May they be enabled to live more effectively with pain.

The pain-control methods described in this book are *not* meant to replace the expert help that only a physician or other qualified health-care professional can provide to pain patients. They should therefore be used in consultation with such a person.

If you are suffering from a chronic-pain condition, I wish you God's healing and grace.

Siang-Yang Tan, Ph.D.
Arcadia, California

Part One
Clinical Pain

1

Pain: Problem,
Puzzle or Gift?

P
AIN HAS BEEN DESCRIBED AS "ONE OF THE MOST CHALLENGING
problems in medicine and biology."[1]
Pain is a challenge to the person suffering from it, to the
health-care professional treating pain patients, to the scientist or researcher trying to better understand pain and its mechanisms, and to
society itself, which must use whatever resources are available in attempting to prevent or alleviate pain.

Almost everyone has experienced pain at some time or other, but
pain is difficult to define precisely. Even scientists and health-care
professionals do not always agree on the exact meaning of the word.

One technical definition of pain that has been proposed by the
International Association for the Study of Pain (IASP) reads as follows: "Pain is an unpleasant sensory and emotional experience associated with actual or potential tissue damage, or described in terms of
such damage."[2] Even this definition is not fully satisfactory. Drs. Ronald Melzack and Patrick Wall have suggested that pain can best be
viewed as a *category* of experiences that have several sensory or physical *and* affective or emotional dimensions. In other words, both physically noxious and emotionally negative components need to be pres-

ent for an experience to be described as pain.

However we define pain, it is a very real problem for literally billions of people around the world. Estimates vary on the number of Americans suffering from chronic pain conditions of various sorts that last over an extended period of time, but Dr. John Bonica has stated that chronic pain afflicts about 30 percent of Americans. Around one-half to two-thirds of these chronic pain sufferers are partially or totally disabled for days, weeks or months, some of them even permanently.[3]

Drs. Wayne and Charles Oates have estimated that some 90 million Americans experience chronic pain.[4] Dr. Thomas Miller has stated that about 65 million Americans suffer from chronic pain and that more than 700 million work days are lost annually in the U.S. as a result of chronic pain conditions. Together with health-care costs, these lost days represent almost $60 billion a year.[5] Dr. Richard Sternbach places the cost of chronic pain to our economy even higher, close to an appalling $80 billion annually![6]

When all pain complaints were considered, whether short-term acute or long-term chronic, a study over a three-year period by the National Center for Health Statistics found that pain was the major complaint in 70 million physician visits, of which 10 million were for back pain, resulting in over 4 billion lost work days, of which one-third were for low back pain. In addition, tens of millions in the U.S. are affected by chronic pain like arthritis and migraine headaches.[7]

The Nuprin Pain Report, the first national survey on pain in the United States, was commissioned by the Bristol-Myers Company, the distributors of Nuprin, and conducted by Louis Harris & Associates, a national survey research organization, in consultation with Dr. Richard Sternbach, a world-renowned psychologist in the area of pain treatment. The survey found in 1985 that 98 percent of all patient complaints of pain consisted of the following major pain conditions: headache, backache, muscle and joint pain, stomach pain, menstrual cycle pain, dental pain. Back pain was the single most common source of pain, especially of chronic pain.[8]

Chronic Pain and You

Such statistics are of little comfort to you if you are suffering from a painful condition or know of someone who is. However, they do underscore how common pain is, and they point out the need to understand and deal with pain more effectively.

Pain is viewed as a *problem* for the majority of people suffering from it—especially chronic pain conditions that last over a period of time, usually for at least several months, up to several years or even permanently. As such, pain is seen to be negative, destructive, unhelpful and even as an "evil" to be mastered, controlled, reduced and if possible even eliminated. The *problem* of pain from this perspective therefore requires methods or interventions for pain control. Subsequent chapters in this book will discuss such options.

Pain is also a *puzzle* or mystery that we have not fully figured out to date. There is much about the experience or perception of pain and its underlying biological, psychological, cultural, interpersonal and spiritual dimensions that we do not yet understand. Drs. Melzack and Wall have pointed out that the link between physical injury and pain is a variable one: pain is not always directly proportional to the extent of tissue damage or injury. There are at least four reasons for this conclusion.

First, *there can be injury without pain,* as in the case of people who have a congenital insensitivity to pain—who are born without the ability to feel pain. Second, *there can be pain without injury.* Tension headaches are a common example of pain without obvious injury. Third, *there can be pain that is disproportionate to the severity or extent of injury,* as with the excruciating pain often experienced by people in the passing of kidney stones. Finally, *there can be pain that persists even after the healing of injury,* as in the case of "phantom limb" pain where, after the amputation of a limb, a person still experiences intense pain in the limb that no longer exists.[9]

All these examples provided by Melzack and Wall point to the variable link or relationship between injury or tissue damage and the pain that is eventually experienced by the individual, emphasizing the *complexity* of the pain experience, and hence the *puzzle* of pain as a phenomenon that requires further research and study as well as better and more sophisticated theories to explain its mechanisms and multiple dimensions. The next chapter will deal with the puzzle of pain and understanding pain in more detail.

Finally, pain has also paradoxically been viewed as a *gift*. A recent book by world-renowned Christian surgeon Dr. Paul Brand, who has spent much of his life and ministry helping leprosy patients, and writer Philip Yancey is entitled *Pain: The Gift Nobody Wants*.[10] It contains a warning that life without pain could really hurt you. Based on his work as a hand surgeon in India that resulted in a number of significant breakthroughs in the treatment of leprosy, Dr. Brand concluded that the simple loss of pain sensation or the ability to experience pain caused most of the ravages of leprosy, like open ulcers, missing fingers and toes, and blindness. Patients with this disease were destroying themselves because they had lost the *gift* of pain.

People born without the ability to feel pain or with a congenital insensitivity to pain are further examples pointing to the value of pain. Brand therefore advocates a greater acceptance of pain as a necessary part of our lives. And he emphasizes the need for each one of us to learn how to make pain a friend and crucial ally in medical treatment as well as in true health. Pain can serve as a gift or ally in warning us of more serious physical problems or helping us to grow spiritually and emotionally. We can therefore learn to cope with or even to triumph in pain and to view it as a gift from God for our ultimate well-being. In this sense, there is some good in pain.

Whether we view pain as a *problem* to be overcome, a *puzzle* to be solved or a *gift* to be thankful for, pain is certainly a challenge. As a complex experience consisting of both sensory, or physical, and emotional dimensions, the challenge of pain actually requires us to view it as a problem, a puzzle *and* a gift!

If you suffer from pain or know someone who does, this book has been written to help you understand how it is possible to cope more effectively with pain—to better manage chronic pain from a Christian perspective. The following chapters will provide you with practical methods for pain control and Christian perspectives on healing and the power of God, as well as on suffering and the grace of God.

2

Understanding Pain

T HE FIRST STEP IN LEARNING TO MANAGE CHRONIC PAIN EFFEC-
tively is to have some understanding of pain itself. We have not
achieved a complete understanding of pain to date; there is
much about it that we still do not comprehend. But our knowledge
of pain and its mechanisms—what it is, how it occurs—contains more
pieces to the puzzle of pain than we have ever had before. The area
of pain research continues to be an exciting and quickly developing
one.

If you are suffering from a chronic-pain condition, you already
know about pain from firsthand experience. Some of the material in
this chapter is quite technical or clinical, but it may still be helpful for
you to read it through for a clearer understanding of pain. However,
you may also choose to skip the first part of this chapter and go on
to the section called "The Psychology of Pain."

Theories of Pain

In order to understand pain more fully, we need to begin with the
major theories of pain. The traditional and earlier theory of pain was
first proposed by the seventeenth-century philosopher Descartes. His

view was that pain is produced by a direct pain transmission system in the body—a system that carries pain messages or signals from receptors in body areas with tissue injury or damage to a pain center in the brain. Hence, he saw pain primarily as a specific physical sensation with intensity directly proportional to the extent of tissue injury or damage.

In this view, the greater the extent of injury, the worse the pain will be. If you accidentally hit your finger lightly with a hammer, you should experience less pain than if you accidentally hit your finger very hard with a hammer. This traditional specificity view or theory of pain has been around for a long time and still affects the way we think about pain. However, upon closer reflection and upon observation of actual pain experiences reported, it becomes clear that Descartes's theory is too simple—it is inadequate and inaccurate for understanding pain in all of its complexity.

In the previous chapter, the variable and inconsistent link between injury and pain was pointed out, with a few brief examples. Pain therefore cannot be viewed simply as a specific physical sensation in direct proportion to the degree of injury or tissue damage, although this view is true to a certain extent. For example, we often do experience greater pain when we have a large laceration on our knees than when we have a small cut. But this direct relationship between pain and extent of injury does not always hold up.

In addition to the examples already mentioned in chapter one, a particularly well-known report of different experiences of pain from similar conditions of physical injury or tissue damage was provided by Dr. H. K. Beecher, a researcher in the late 1940s and 1950s. He studied the behavior of soldiers severely wounded in battle during World War II, then compared it to what he later observed in a group of civilians who had surgical wounds similar to those sustained by the soldiers.

His findings were dramatic and somewhat astonishing: only one out of three wounded soldiers wanted morphine for his pain, whereas four out of five of the civilians with surgical wounds complained of having severe pain and asked for morphine. In other words, about 65 percent of soldiers severely wounded in battle but only 20 percent of civilians with similar wounds associated with major surgery reported having little or no pain.[1]

Dr. Beecher therefore concluded that such data did not support the common belief that wounds are always associated with pain, and the greater the wound or injury, the worse the pain. Rather, his findings indicated that there is no simple direct relationship between the wound or injury per se and the pain experienced. Beecher attempted to explain his results by pointing out that the *significance* or *meaning* of the wound determines to a great extent the pain experienced.

For the wounded soldier, the wound usually meant the end of fighting and the prospect of being sent home alive from the battle-field. Therefore, the typical response included relief, thankfulness, even euphoria. However, for the civilian recovering from similar surgical wounds, the major surgery and associated wounds usually meant physical disability and a future full of uncertainty and possible calamity. Therefore, the typical response included depression, anxiety or worry—and a greater perception of pain.

As a result of dissatisfaction with Descartes's original specificity theory of pain, several other researchers, such as Goldscheider in the late 1800s, Livingston in 1943 and Noordenbos in 1959, proposed alternative theories of pain that gave greater attention to the role of the spinal cord in modulating or coordinating the pain signals coming from the peripheral areas of the body before sending them on to the brain. Such "patterns of pain messages" were eventually transmitted on to brain centers that registered pain, and so these revised views were together categorized as the "pattern theory" of pain.

While these revised views did not assert that pain was directly proportional to the extent of injury or wounds, they were still somewhat vague, and they did not explain how pain could also be controlled or influenced by the brain itself, since the brain was still viewed as a passive receiver of pain messages.[2]

The Gate-Control Theory

A more exciting and helpful theory of pain was proposed in 1965 by Melzack and Wall, going beyond both specificity and pattern theories of pain. It is called the *gate-control theory of pain.*[3] It can be briefly summarized as consisting of the following five major propositions:

1. The transmission of nerve impulses or messages from the peripheral parts of the body to the spinal cord is controlled by a spinal gating mechanism in the dorsal horn of the spinal cord, especially in the *substantia gelatinosa* area. This spinal-cord "pain gate" can close or open its gates to nerve impulses or messages arriving in this area and thereby stop them or pass them on to other nerve networks that carry these messages eventually to the brain as pain messages.

2. The spinal pain gate is influenced by the relative amount of activity in large-diameter and small-diameter nerve fibers. The pain gate tends to close when large fibers are activated, while activity in small fibers tends to open the pain gate.

3. The spinal pain gate is also influenced by nerve impulses that descend from the brain itself. The brain is no longer seen only as a receiver of pain messages but also as an active contributor of messages to the pain gate in the spinal cord.

4. A specialized system of large, rapidly conducting nerve fibers (called the central control trigger) activates specific thinking processes in the brain that can then influence the spinal pain gate by way of nerve fibers that descend to it.

5. Pain is eventually experienced only if the spinal pain gate is relatively open after the various nerve messages are processed and then allowed to go on to the brain, where they are finally interpreted as pain messages.

In simpler terms, the gate-control theory of pain states that *information reaches the brain only if the pain gate is open.* The balance of activity in large or small fibers that go up to the brain (large fibers tend to close the gate while small ones tend to open it) and in fibers that descend from the higher centers in the brain determines whether the pain gate is relatively open or closed.

In recent years, there has been more emphasis on pain gates in the brain itself. Most recently, Melzack has proposed an even more sophisticated new theory of brain function that emphasizes how the widespread large network of neurons in the brain is spatially distributed and linked together, first by genetics and later molded by sensory inputs or experience. He calls this network, which serves as the anatomical foundation of a unified sense of "body-self," a *neuromatrix*. He asserts that the brain does not just passively receive and analyze sensory inputs. Instead, the brain actually actively produces perceptual experiences, including pain, even when there are no external inputs present. Therefore, phantom-limb pain—pain experienced in a limb that is now absent—is no longer a mystery: in Melzack's neuromatrix theory, *the brain itself* generates or produces the experience of the body and therefore can cause phantom-limb pain. A particular part of the brain called the *limbic system*, where emotions are processed, may play a crucial role in all of this. Such a theory has begun to stimulate new and exciting research programs to further our understanding of brain function, including pain perception or experience and how to better control pain.[4]

The gate-control theory of pain also emphasizes that pain is a complex experience consisting of at least three major dimensions: *thinking* ("cognitive-evaluative"), *emotional or feeling* ("motivational-affective") and *physical* ("sensory-discriminative") dimensions. In other words, what we are thinking or saying to ourselves and how we are feeling emotionally can directly affect our ultimate pain experience. The physical, or sensory, dimension usually related to injury or tissue damage is only part of the story.

The gate-control theory has resulted in many new methods for pain control, in addition to the traditional ones of taking pain medications or having surgery. Later chapters in this book will describe such methods for pain control, some of which may be helpful to you or someone you know who may be suffering from pain.

The Pathways of Pain

Apparently there are two major nerve pathways or routes that messages of injury can travel from the peripheral receptors of the body to the brain itself. The first pathway is called the *paleospinothalamic tract*. It courses through the center of the spinal cord onto the part of the midbrain called the thalamus. There are many connections among the nerve fibers of this major pathway, and the signals or messages conducted along it to the brain travel relatively slowly. If such injury signals or messages are registered in the brain itself as pain, the pain is often not clearly localized and tends to be a deep, burning, aching type of pain.

The second major pathway by which injury messages in the spinal cord are conveyed to the brain is called the *neospinothalamic tract*. This route is more efficient, capable of carrying more information more quickly to the brain. This pathway has fewer connections among its nerve fibers. If the injury signals are eventually experienced as pain in the brain areas, the pain is usually sharp and intense and is more clearly localized.[5]

However, as Melzack has pointed out, so-called "pain pathways" are actually more complex than the descriptions provided, because there are also descending fibers and multiple interconnections, or complex networks, throughout the central nervous system. Hence, his neuromatrix theory of brain function emphasizes *the great influence of the brain itself* in the regulation of perceptual experiences, including pain.

Injury messages or signals in and of themselves do not necessarily register as pain when they arrive at higher centers in the brain. Whether pain is eventually experienced depends on whether the pain gate is relatively open or closed—and there may be pain gates in higher centers of the brain, not just in the spinal cord.

The Chemistry of Pain

One exciting development in the area of pain research in recent decades has been the discovery, in some parts of the brain, of certain pain-suppressing chemicals or substances that seem to act in ways similar to powerful drugs such as narcotics or morphine. Some examples of these chemicals are *endorphins, enkephalins* (enkephalin is actually a type of endorphin) and *dynorphin.* The nervous system apparently has its own natural analgesics or painkillers that come into play when pain is experienced and pain control is needed. These substances, when released, may play a crucial role in closing the pain gate (or gates).

Richard Sternbach has pointed out that there is another possible pain-gate control process that involves a different chemical, *serotonin.* Serotonin plays a variety of roles in different parts of the body; in the brain it seems to be crucial for sleep and for emotional balance. When there is a depletion or decrease in serotonin, insomnia or difficulty in falling asleep and emotional depression often occur—and possibly a decrease in pain tolerance as well. Medications that tend to increase serotonin activity in the brain have been effective in helping patients with chronic pain syndrome reduce insomnia, depression and even pain severity.[6]

The Psychology of Pain

Whatever the physiological or biochemical bases of pain may be, research has shown that psychological and social factors also play a key role in pain experience and response. A number of psychosocial factors have been found to influence pain perception. They include ethnic background, socioeconomic status, family size, birth order, present circumstances, meaning of the situation or even of the pain itself (as in Beecher's findings mentioned earlier), anxiety or uncertainty, expectation, depression or hopelessness, and stress. Anxiety, for example, can worsen or even produce pain. In general, moderate levels of arousal tend to increase pain, whereas less intensive or extreme arousal levels tend to reduce pain.[7]

Melzack has stressed therefore that pain is a perceptual experience that is affected by the unique past history of the person experiencing pain, his or her state of mind at the moment, and the meaning he or she gives to the pain-producing situation. For example, if a person has grown up in a family or culture that is very sensitive to pain and therefore has developed a relatively lower tolerance for pain, and if this person is presently anxious, with a tendency to interpret painful experiences as terrible and catastrophic ("the end of the world"), then he or she will end up experiencing the painful situation as more painful. Someone else from a family or culture that is less sensitive to pain, who is relatively relaxed and not as negative or catastrophic about pain may end up experiencing the same painful situation as less painful.

Ellen Catalano, who served as a biofeedback therapist in the pain management center at the University of Virginia Medical Center, has pointed out that the person in chronic pain can have his or her pain affected adversely or positively by his or her environment, including family, previous medical history, possible compensation, job history, cultural expectations, current medical treatments available and other environmental factors.[8]

Before ending this chapter, let me define a few more pain terms that will be used throughout this book, so that you can more easily follow the chapters to come. These pain terms include: *pain threshold* and *pain tolerance, experimental* and *clinical pain,* and *acute* and *chronic pain.*[9]

Pain Threshold and Pain Tolerance

Pain threshold is the term usually used to refer to the point at which one first perceives a stimulus as painful. *Pain tolerance* is the term usually used to refer to the point at which one is not willing to accept noxious stimulation of a higher degree or magnitude or to continue to endure such stimulation at a given level. Pain threshold is generally related more to physiological conditions, whereas pain tolerance appears to be more affected by emotional or psychological factors.

Experimental and Clinical Pain

Experimental pain refers to pain that is induced in laboratory studies by the use of a number of noxious stimuli such as heat, pressure, ice water and electric shock. For example, an individual may be asked to put his or her hand in ice-cold water and then to indicate when he or she first experiences the water as painful (pain threshold level) and when he or she cannot take the pain any longer (pain tolerance level). In this example, the measurement is in terms of minutes and seconds of hand immersion in the ice-cold water.

Clinical pain refers to pain experienced as a result of real-life pain, usually but not necessarily as a result of some tissue damage or injury. Examples of clinical, real-life pain include migraine and tension headaches, low-back pain, arthritic pain, abdominal pain, and pain due to injuries such as cuts, fractures and burns.

There are obvious differences between experimental pain and clinical pain. For example, experimental pain caused by laboratory pain stressors is usually experienced as less threatening or less anxiety-provoking, more specific and identifiable, of shorter duration or time-limited—and it can be ended or terminated at will. Laboratory studies of pain-control methods using experimental pain stressors cannot, therefore, generalize their findings to clinical pain until further research studies are done with people with real-life, clinical-pain conditions. This book is concerned with *clinical pain*, especially of the chronic type, although studies using experimental pain will be cited where helpful or useful.

Acute and Chronic Pain

Acute pain refers to pain of limited duration, normally defined as lasting six months or less. It is typically an alarm or signal to the body that there has been some tissue damage or injury requiring immediate attention. In this sense, acute pain can be seen as a gift.

Chronic pain, on the other hand, refers to pain that has lasted more than six months in duration. As Sternbach has pointed out, unlike acute pain, chronic pain is usually *not* a symptom, not a warning signal and not a need for rest. In other words, the difference between acute and chronic pain is not only a matter of duration. Sternbach has put it this way:

> Chronic pain is a syndrome composed of a number of physical, emotional and behavioral changes which can convert otherwise healthy individuals into invalids. Chronic pain is like a "false alarm"—a warning signal that serves no purpose. In its effect on the individual who has it and on the family, chronic pain is very like a debilitating disease.[10]

Chronic pain can be further divided into three major subcategories as suggested by Drs. Turk, Meichenbaum and Genest, well-known psychologists in the cognitive-behavioral treatment of pain: *chronic recurrent pain,* with periods of intense pain alternating with periods without pain, from an apparently benign condition that is not worsening (e.g., tension and migraine headaches); *chronic intractable-benign pain,* where there is persistent pain varying in intensity but with no pain-free periods, also from a benign or nonmalignant condition (e.g., low-back pain); and *chronic progressive pain,* where the pain is persistent and usually becomes more intense as the organic condition underlying the pain gets progressively worse (e.g., cancer or rheumatoid arthritis).[11]

Measuring Pain

Whether one experiences acute pain or chronic pain of some type, there is a need to measure or describe the pain so that we can better understand it as well as evaluate the effectiveness of pain-control methods for reducing such pain. *Pain assessment or measurement* has made some significant advances in recent years.[12] Briefly, in addition to experimental pain stressors used to assess pain threshold and tolerance levels, there are three other major categories of pain measurement methods: *behavioral* measures, such as ratings of actual pain behavior or amount of analgesic or pain medication used; *physiological* measures, such as evoked potentials or changes in brain wave activity as shown by an electroencephalogram (EEG) in response to a specific stimulus or by electromyograph (EMG) recordings of muscle tension; and *self-report* measures of subjective pain experiences made by the person who is having pain, such as verbal or visual analogue scales of pain intensity, as with the McGill Pain Questionnaire developed by Ronald Melzack, which is the most widely used self-rating pain questionnaire today.[13]

A simple verbal pain intensity rating scale that you can use to rate your subjective experience of pain is a 0-10 point scale of pain intensity as follows: 0—No Pain at All; 5—Moderate Pain; 10—Excruciating Pain. The higher the number you choose, the more intense the pain you are experiencing.

A visual analogue scale of pain intensity is simply a line drawn between two extreme points, one representing no pain at all and the other the worst possible pain. You simply put an *X* on this line wherever you feel your pain is best represented visually and spatially.

You can also use the following overall measure of Present Pain Intensity from the McGill Pain Questionnaire, using a 0-5 point scale as follows: 0—No Pain; 1—Mild Pain; 2—Discomforting Pain; 3—Distressing Pain; 4—Horrible Pain; and 5—Excruciating Pain. This pain intensity scale (0-5) is similar to the 0-10 point scale mentioned earlier. You can use either of these simple, straightforward self-report scales of pain intensity to rate your subjective pain experience, whether acute or chronic, and to help you keep track daily of your progress in pain management.

In the following chapters of this book I will be describing the major methods for pain control that are available today. Mastering or overcoming pain, especially chronic pain, is a valid goal, but learning to live with and manage pain is equally important for the many chronic-pain sufferers who have found no easy answers so far to their struggle with pain.

While we must not make pain into a virtue or even a god (for example, by glorifying pain as a special blessing from God that we should continue to hang on to)—because it is not that—God can at times use pain in our lives for good. He can speak to us, warn us, discipline us or help us grow through experiences of pain in our lives—always giving us his grace that is sufficient for our every need (2 Cor 12:9-10). However, he can also manifest his healing power in answer to prayer for healing of painful conditions. A biblical perspective on healing in the context of pain will be provided later in this book.

3

Medical & Surgical
Methods
for Pain Control

BOB IS A THIRTY-TWO-YEAR-OLD INSURANCE SALES REPRESENTATIVE who has been working very hard in his profession for almost a decade. He has been in his present job ever since he graduated from college with a degree in business studies. He has done very well and has been a top salesperson in his company for several years now. However, he has to work long and late hours, often on weekends as well. He makes very good money and has managed to purchase his own home in a nice suburb of the city, as well as an expensive, fun-to-drive sports car.

In the past year, Bob has been experiencing low-back pain. It started when he tried to lift a heavy box in his garage at home during the Christmas holidays a year ago. He was about twenty pounds overweight then and had not been exercising regularly or keeping fit for a couple of years, mainly due to his hectic work schedule.

Bob's low-back pain has actually worsened over the past year. Initially he tried to deal with it by resting for a few days. However, it got worse, and he began to experience intense and at times excruciating pain in his lower back region. He therefore consulted his physician early in the new year. His physician prescribed a number of medications, including some pain medication, after x-rays did not reveal any obvious physical damage or injury. He was also told to take bed rest for a few days.

Bob's pain improved somewhat, and he was able to return to work after taking another week off. However, as his work schedule became hectic and very demanding again, his back pain returned, sometimes with great intensity. A few months later he attempted to lift something in his office one day and experienced excruciating pain in his back. He almost couldn't straighten up. He went to the doctor that very day.

After prescribing some more pain medications, the doctor referred him this time to an orthopedic surgeon who specialized in low-back pain and back injuries. Although further diagnostic tests—including an MRI—did not yield any clear-cut nerve or disc damage, surgery was discussed as another possible treatment option.

Bob took a few months to consider surgery because he did not want to rush into such a drastic treatment. But his low-back pain continued to recur, and now almost a year had gone by.

Bob's pain condition has become a chronic one. Out of desperation, he has decided to see the orthopedic surgeon again and seriously consider surgery as his next option. Yet he still has some reservations and mixed feelings because he recently read about the low success rates of such surgery for low-back pain in general (except for clear-cut cases of a protruding lumbar disc compromising or impinging upon a nerve root), as well as its many negative side effects.

A Common Ailment
The above scenario is not uncommon. Low-back pain is one of the most frequently occurring conditions of chronic pain, and the Nuprin Pain Report actually found back pain to be the single most prevalent source of pain, particularly chronic pain.

Dr. Richard Hanson and Dr. Kenneth Gerber, two psychologists involved in the treatment of pain patients, have pointed out that low-back pain is the most common cause of workdays missed due to pain-related disability, especially for people between the ages of 18 and 44. They also cited the Nuprin study, which reveals that 14 percent of all adults in the United States have serious chronic back pain conditions, while approximately 14 percent more have less severe back pain that nevertheless still interferes with their daily work or routine.[1] Drs. Hanson and Gerber note that surgery for low-back pain problems has had poor success in general, despite the fact that about 400,000 surgeries were performed in 1986 alone for lumbar disc disease. There is apparently much diagnostic confusion when dealing with low-back pain patients.[2]

What pain control methods or treatments are available for someone like Bob with chronic low-back pain or any chronic pain condition? According to Melzack and Wall, there are presently four major approaches to pain control and the relief of suffering: (1) *pharmacological* (drugs/medications), (2) *surgical,* (3) *sensory modulation of input* (e.g., nerve blocks, transcutaneous electrical nerve stimulation or TENS, physical therapy, massage and manipulation, heat therapy, acupuncture) and (4) *psychological* (e.g., relaxation techniques, calming self-talk, pleasant imagery, cognitive coping skills, cognitive therapy methods, stress-inoculation training, modeling, biofeedback, hypnosis, operant conditioning or reinforcement methods, pacing and pleasurable activities, psychotherapy, marital and/or family therapy, support groups).[3] I would add a fifth category that falls somewhat within the psychological but transcends it, and that is the *spiritual,* including prayer for healing; faith in God and his Word, the Bible, that gives meaning and hope in the midst of suffering and pain; and the support of the church and the Christian community.

It is important to differentiate between *pain* and *suffering.* Some people who experience pain may not suffer much emotionally or spiritually because they are able to cope with their pain or experience hope and meaning in the midst of it. Others who experience pain of even relatively mild intensity may nevertheless suffer much more emotionally and spiritually. Dr. Eric Cassel has noted that people in pain often report suffering from the pain when

☐ they feel out of control
☐ the origin or source of the pain is unknown
☐ the pain is overwhelming or chronic
☐ the meaning of the pain is negative

Conversely, suffering can be reduced, even if the pain persists, by

☐ making known the origin or source of the pain
☐ changing the meaning of the pain into a more constructive one
☐ showing that it can be controlled and that an end to the pain is possible soon[4]

Dr. Cassel emphasizes that people in pain often perceive pain as a threat not only to their physical well-being or their very lives but also to their integrity or intactness as persons. He therefore defines suffering as "the state of severe distress associated with events that threaten the intactness of the person."[5]

Pain is only one of such possible events. Pain and suffering are definitely related, but they are not synonymous or identical. While this book focuses on pain control, it will also deal with the larger issue of coping with suffering associated with pain.

In the rest of this chapter, I will describe briefly the major *pharmacological* and *surgical* approaches to pain control. If you are experiencing a chronic pain condition, you should consult your physician or surgeon and discuss such treatment options thoroughly with him or her before proceeding with any of them.

Pain Medications and Drugs

The pharmacological or chemical control of pain through the use of various pain medications or drugs is one of the first methods people in pain use for alleviation of their pain. Melzack and Wall have categorized the drugs that relieve pain without causing a loss of consciousness into the following major groups: (1) the mild analgesics, including aspirin and acetaminophen; (2) the more powerful analgesics—the opiates (or narcotics)—that derive from morphine; (3) the opioid compounds that are structurally like morphine but are not derived from it; (4) psychotropic drugs; and (5) inhalant drugs such as nitrous oxide.[6]

Aspirin and other Non-Steroidal Anti-Inflammatory Drugs (NSAIDs). This remarkable category of pain medications includes aspirin (acetylsalicylic acid) and other salicylates, as well as other NSAIDs such as indomethacin (Indocin), mefenamic acid (Ponstel), ibuprofen (Advil, Motrin, Nuprin), piroxicam (Feldene) and others. These medications have three main therapeutic actions: against pain, against inflammation and against fever. The specific drugs vary in their relative power to produce such results and also in their side effects. The best known nonprescription, over-the-counter medications in this category are aspirin and ibuprofen.

These pain medications are often used for pain associated with injuries such as a broken leg or bruised skin or pain conditions like headaches, low-back pain and arthritic joint pain. The site of action of these medications seems to be on the injured area itself and not on peripheral nerves or on the central nervous system. Apparently, pain that is the result of events which do not lead to inflammatory reactions does not respond much to these drugs. They do, unfortunately, have some side effects. Aspirin in particular can cause gastric irritation and bleeding, although a special coating on the aspirin tablets can reduce such side effects significantly. Overdoses can also affect the brain, liver, kidney and blood chemistry.

Acetaminophen. Acetaminophen, another mild analgesic, is now more widely used because of the potentially serious side effects of aspirin in people who have gastric disorders. It is the second most popular mild analgesic and is sold under brand names such as Tylenol and Panadol. It has no significant anti-inflammatory actions, unlike aspirin and other NSAIDs. It is therefore less effective for arthritis, skin injuries and other pain conditions involving major inflammation of peripheral tissues, including blood vessels. Liver and kidney damage are possible serious side effects of high doses of acetaminophen. It is, however, easier on the stomach than aspirin.

Opiates (narcotics). This group of pain medications called *opiates* or *narcotics* includes compounds such as opium (which contains morphine and smaller amounts of other alkaloids like codeine and thebaine) and other synthetic ones, for example, heroin, hydromorphone (Dilaudid), oxymorphone (Numorphan), oxycodone and dihydrocodone. They all produce analgesia, or pain relief, and at higher doses they can cause drowsiness, mood changes and mental clouding. The site of their analgesic effects is clearly in the central nervous system.

Narcotics can be administered by mouth, by injection, even intravenously if very rapid action is needed. They are used most frequently in emergencies with quick onset of intense pain. They are often injected or given intravenously for severe injuries, heart attacks and abdominal crises. They are also employed to control pain after surgery, childbirth or labor pain, and pain associated with terminal disease such as cancer. Narcotics are often used—and sometimes abused, when administered too freely—for other chronic pain conditions like migraine and other headache pain and low-back pain. For example, oxycodone is frequently used in combination with aspirin (as Percodan) or acetaminophen (as Percocet), and hydrocodone in combination with acetaminophen (as Vicodin or Tylenol #3).

A serious concern with narcotics or opiates is possible addiction to them. However, the danger of addiction has often been overstated. As Melzack and Wall have pointed out, more nonsense on narcotic addiction is written by both physicians and the popular press than on any other medical issue. An unfortunate consequence has been the tendency to undermedicate patients with severe pain conditions who may appropriately need higher doses of narcotics for adequate and humane pain control. Narcotics also have side effects such as constipation and nausea.

Synthetic opioids. Pharmaceutical companies have tried to produce synthetic variations of narcotic analgesic drugs that minimize unwanted side effects, while maintaining or improving the desired pain-relieving effects. They have done so in three main ways. First, they modified the poppy plant molecules to produce synthetic opioids such as heroin, hydromorphone and hydrocodone. Second, they developed purely synthetic drugs that have narcotic effects, for example, meperidine (Demerol), fentanyl, methadone (Dolophine), and propoxyphene (Darvon). Finally, they tried to produce variants of the newly discovered endogenous narcotics found in the human body (endorphins, dynorphins and enkephalins). The large molecular size of the dynorphins and endorphins makes synthesis difficult. Pharmacologists have worked more on the enkephalins, which are short-chain peptides, and produced a synthetic compound called DADL (D-alamine-D-leucine enkephalin). Several synthetic opioids are therefore now available for use as analgesic medications.

Psychotropic drugs. Psychotropic drugs are usually used for their effects on psychological functions such as mood. The three main psychotropic medications are antidepressants, major tranquilizers, and antianxiety drugs or minor tranquilizers. It should be pointed out that such powerful psychotropic drugs have therapeutic as well as unwanted side effects. People with chronic pain often develop depression as a result of their experiencing persistent pain. Antidepressant drugs have been found to be effective for treating the depression as well as the pain itself.

Melzack and Wall noted that recent research has shown that the tricyclic antidepressants in particular have analgesic effects. For example, imipramine (Tofranil) has been found to be effective for reducing chronic osteoarthritic and rheumatoid arthritis pain, and amitryptyline (Elavil) for reducing pain in migraine and chronic tension headaches.

The major tranquilizers, especially the phenothiazines, such as fluphenazine (Prolixin) and methotrimeprazine (Levoprome), are also used at times alone or together with the antidepressants to treat a number of different types of pain. However, minor tranquilizers or antianxiety drugs such as the benzodiazepines (such as diazepam or Valium and chlordiazepoxide or Librium) have not been found to be effective for chronic pain control and may even increase depression and pain in the long run. Yet they can have some short-term effects in relieving muscle pain and spasm and such anxiety-related disorders as irritable bowel syndrome.

Combination analgesics. A number of pain medications have been combined for increased effectiveness in pain control. Aspirin is frequently used together with small doses of codeine, with much greater analgesic effect than either drug alone. Another effective combination is a mild narcotic with a low dose of a tricyclic antidepressant. Patients with severe cancer pain have found two other combination analgesics to be especially powerful: morphine with dextro-amphetamine, and methadone with amitriptyline and a nonnarcotic analgesic.

Inhalant analgesics. A mixture of nitrous oxide and oxygen that can be inhaled through a mask has been found to be effective for a variety of pain conditions (without loss of consciousness) including postoperative pain, labor pain, pain due to heart attack, cancer pain that is intermittent or spasmodic, pain due to dental procedures, and pain due to injuries usually seen in hospital emergency departments. Melzack and Wall advocate using such a relatively safe mixture of nitrous oxide and oxygen as inhalant analgesics for noxious or painful medical procedures such as bone taps, spinal punctures, and injections into the lymphatic system.

Drugs like nitrous oxide in large quantities function more like anesthetics, producing unconsciousness, but in smaller quantities they can have analgesic effects without loss of consciousness.

Other drugs that may be prescribed for pain control include *steroid hormones,* which are very powerful anti-inflammatory substances and may be needed in injuries causing much inflammation, but which also tend to weaken a crucial body defense mechanism such that infections may occur. And there are other specific medications, like those which partially inhibit the sympathetic nervous system and hence can be used to reduce pain due to injury to the sympathetic nerves, and medications used mainly as anticonvulsants for epilepsy (e.g., carbamazepine or Tegretol), which may also be helpful for pain control in patients with certain neuralgias.

A well-known example is *trigeminal neuralgia* (or *tic douloureux*), an excruciatingly painful condition involving the nerves of the head and face, characterized by paroxysmal attacks of severe pain that may occur spontaneously or be triggered by behaviors like chewing, eating or talking.[7] *Muscle relaxants* such as carisoprodol (Soma), cyclobenzaprine (Flexeril), methocarbamol (Robaxin) and orphenadrine citrate (Norflex) may also be used, for a short period of up to a few weeks, to treat muscle pain due to persistently contracted, tense muscle fibers.[8]

In a recent book on the prevention and treatment of all types of headaches, Dr. Frank Minirth, a well-known Christian psychiatrist, listed the following available drugs or medications that can be used, mainly for migraine headaches or pain: *nonprescription (over-the-counter) drugs* such as aspirin or salicylates, ibuprofens and acetaminophens; and *prescription drugs* such as narcotics (codeine, morphine, Demerol, Percodan, Vicodin), ergotamines, ergotamines plus caffeine, antidepressants, beta blockers, prednisone, Sumatriptan, minor tranquilizers and combination medicines.[9]

It is obvious therefore that control of pain through drugs or medications is widely practiced and available. Unfortunately, analgesics or pain medications are not always effective for pain control, especially for people suffering from certain chronic pain conditions, like Bob with his low-back pain. Medications should be used wisely and carefully and, for prescription drugs, always under the supervision of a physician.

If medications seem to be necessary in controlling your pain, it is advisable to follow some guidelines for the proper use of analgesics or pain medications as recommended by Sternbach.[10]

First, remember that while analgesics are powerful and helpful for acute pain, especially for those recovering from surgery or injury, they are not as helpful for those who have chronic pain conditions. In fact, in the long run, using pain medications—particularly narcotics, which are potentially addictive—can and often does cause *more* problems for the person with chronic pain. *Tolerance* to narcotics is a biological fact: the more and longer you take them, the more you'll need in order to continue having pain relief because your liver produces enzymes to neutralize the effects of the narcotics. Over time, *dependence* and possibly *addiction* develop. Dependence is manifested when, once the use of narcotics is stopped suddenly after prolonged use, a patient experiences withdrawal symptoms such as tremors, diarrhea and cramps, runny nose and jittery feelings. Some pain patients may even experience a "craving" for the particular drug or drugs and therefore demonstrate a full-blown addiction, although many who are *dependent* on such medications do not experience cravings and thus are not addicted per se to them. It should be pointed out again that while the dangers of narcotic addiction are real, they are not as great as is often claimed.

Second, it is crucial to know that the best way to take analgesics is to follow your physician's instructions and, in the case of over-the-counter medications, to follow the instructions on the label. They usually state something like "take one or two tablets every three to four hours as needed for pain." Many people with chronic pain are ashamed of having to take pain medications and therefore delay their intake until they are in severe pain. By then, they need to take much more or switch to a more potent drug because their pain is so bad, starting a vicious cycle that actually increases subsequent analgesic use. A wiser and better way is to take the pain medications according to a strict time schedule, for example, every four hours or so, and to stick to the recommended dosage, such as one tablet each time. This way, the pain is often kept at a more moderate intensity throughout the day, so that you can generally function although there is some degree of pain. Pain medications for chronic pain should, therefore, generally *not* be taken on an "as needed" basis. They should be taken according to a strict time schedule. The "as-needed" schedule is more appropriate for acute pain situations.

Third, in order to avoid tolerance and dependence, you should try to take the weakest analgesic that is effective in helping you cope with your chronic pain condition. Otherwise you'll be resorting to stronger and more potent pain drugs too soon because of tolerance effects.

Finally, in the long run, for the majority of people suffering from chronic pain conditions it is best to try to quit taking pain medications altogether. They have side effects, and long-term use of them (whether aspirin, ibuprofen, acetaminophen or the stronger narcotics) can have even more adverse effects. Nonprescription analgesics like aspirin can be stopped more suddenly, with little or no ill consequences. Quitting narcotics as pain medications is more complicated—stopping abruptly may lead to a sudden sharp increase in pain as well as often unpleasant withdrawal symptoms. Hence, a more gradual tapering off from narcotics is usually recommended. Make sure you consult your physician and collaborate or cooperate with him or her. You may need to go to a pain clinic or treatment center if you are not able to quit or taper off on your own with your physician's help. Pain treatment centers or clinics will be described in a later chapter of this book. If you have already been on medications for a long time and want to taper off or quit, you'll also need the help of other pain-control methods, especially psychological and spiritual approaches, which will be described in the next few chapters.

Surgical Control of Pain

Surgery or *neurosurgery* is another traditional medical or biological method for pain control that has been used with many pain patients.

Surgery can be very helpful for a number of painful medical conditions that can be corrected by an operation of some sort using the skills of a surgeon. For example, in cases of gall bladder disease, herniated discs in the spinal cord or degenerative disease of a joint, surgery can often correct the underlying problem and therefore relieve the person of pain. Also, in cases of terminal disease such as advanced stages of cancer, where death is imminent and there is considerable widespread pain, *neurosurgery* may be helpful in easing the pain. For example, major nerve pathways in the spinal cord can be cut (cordotomy). Such drastic surgery is effective in the short run, but pain often recurs in the long run, and there are also side effects like serious weakness of the arms and legs and bladder- or bowel-control problems. For terminally ill patients who are near death, such side effects and long-term prognosis for pain control may not be relevant. However, for other chronic-pain patients who are *not* terminally ill, these are important considerations, and hence drastic or invasive surgical control of their chronic pain conditions may not be as attractive or feasible.

Some specific chronic-pain conditions may be helped by surgery, if pain medications or other pain-control methods have not worked. *Trigeminal neuralgia,* mentioned earlier, is one example, where the pain comes from one of the branches of the trigeminal nerve, apparently because of the pulsing of a small artery in the brain as it lies against the nerve. While there are always risks associated with any kind of surgery, at least three types of surgery have been tried with good success on patients with trigeminal neuralgia. *Causalgia* is another example of a pain condition that can possibly benefit from an operation. It refers to a burning pain that is usually due to an injury like a wound or sudden blow that partially damages some sympathetic nerves. A *sympathectomy* or cutting of the sympathetic nerve fibers may be helpful in cases of causalgia. However, as Sternbach rightly points out, neurosurgical control of pain is *not* appropriate for the great majority of chronic pain conditions such as low-back pain, joint pains, headache of all kinds, muscle pains and so on.[11]

In reviewing the major neurosurgical approaches to pain control, Melzack and Wall describe the following procedures: permanent block or destruction of peripheral nerves; surgical or chemical destruction of spinal roots; surgical or chemical destruction of the sympathetic system; cordotomy or the cutting of tracts in the spinal cord; and a number of cerebral or brain operations for the relief of pain, such as mesencephalic tractotomy, thalamotomy, and other cortical lesions. Their conclusion about the effectiveness of neurosurgery or surgical methods for pain control is generally negative. Except for short-term control of pain, especially for terminally ill patients, which can be achieved by performing a cordotomy, they conclude that neurosurgical methods to abolish other forms of chronic pain are often not only unsuccessful but disastrous! They point out that cutting peripheral nerves or nerve fibers in the central nervous system (i.e., in the brain or spinal cord) does not simply stop an input from reaching the brain. Such drastic surgery also has other multiple effects: for example, it permanently changes normal input patterning, it destroys channels that can be useful in controlling pain by sensory-input modulation methods, and it may cause abnormal inputs to the brain as a result of irritating scars and neuromas. Surgical methods for pain control should therefore only be used in exceptional cases where they are clearly warranted. Surgery actually has a pretty dismal, if not disastrous, track record of success in terms of long-term pain relief. Its adverse consequences or side effects are also usually irreversible. Yet over 400,000 operations were performed in 1986 alone for low-back pain conditions!

Fortunately, fewer cordotomies and other drastic neurosurgical procedures are being performed today by neurosurgeons for pain control. They are switching increasingly to more nondestructive methods of pain relief, like the use of devices to electrically stimulate nerves, spinal cord and other specific areas of the brain.[12]

We can be thankful for the availability of pain medications and even surgery for certain types of pain conditions for which they are appropriate and helpful. However, for the majority of people with chronic pain conditions, like Bob, we need to look elsewhere for better pain control methods that do not fail so often or have so many adverse side effects.

4

Sensory Modulation & Other Physical Methods for Pain Control

S ENSORY MODULATION REFERS TO TECHNIQUES THAT MODULATE or influence the sensory input—the amount of physical stimulation allowed to travel through the pain gate in the spinal cord and up to the brain itself. The gate-control theory of pain has had a tremendous impact in this area of sensory-modulation methods for pain control. Four major approaches to the sensory control of pain are suggested by the gate-control theory:

1. The use of anesthetic blocking agents to reduce the number of nerve impulses that travel to the spinal cord area.

2. Low-level stimulation which activates the large fibers that tend to close the spinal pain gate.

3. Intense stimulation which activates brain processes (especially in the brain stem) that send inhibitory nerve messages to the spinal pain gate and other pain gates higher up in the central nervous system, tending to close the pain gates.

4. Direct activation of descending control systems that tend to close the pain gates by using electrical stimulation or pharmaceutical agents

(chemical substances).

Melzack and Wall include the following in their description of sensory-modulation methods for pain control: *temporary local anesthesia;* a number of *physical therapy* techniques practiced by physiatrists (doctors of physical medicine and rehabilitation) and physiotherapists or physical therapists, such as massage and manipulation, heat therapy, and electrical stimulation of nerves, spinal cord and brain; *acupuncture* and other forms of folk medicine; and *hyperstimulation analgesia,* for example, intense transcutaneous electrical stimulation and ice massage.[1] In addition to briefly describing some of these sensory-modulation methods for pain control, this chapter will also cover several other physical methods for pain management such as *exercise, nutrition,* and *sleep and rest.*

Sensory-Modulation Methods for Pain Control

Temporary local anesthesia. The most frequently used method of bringing about temporary local anesthesia is by needle injection of an anesthetic substance or agent into a particular nerve or even a larger general area that needs to be numbed. Dentists do this routinely when they inject a local anesthetic around the area of the teeth they are working on, in order to temporarily numb that area and block out pain as much as possible. Some recent evidence shows that injecting a few milligrams of morphine into the lumbar epidural space can sometimes bring about great pain relief for those experiencing excruciating pain due to spreading cancer in the pelvic area of their bodies, although further research is needed. Morphine is more usually given orally or injected into muscles like the buttock.

Local anesthetic blocks of physical or sensory input can bring about temporary pain relief that can outlast the duration of such blocks. Additional blocks may also lead to further pain reduction of even greater duration. The temporary relief produced may also allow a pain patient to move around a bit more freely, thus further activating the large fibers that can help close the spinal pain gate and facilitate even more pain reduction. There are, however, side effects as well as limitations in the use of temporary local anesthesia as a method of sensory control of pain.

Massage and manipulation. Physical therapy methods for pain control often include massage and manipulation of different sorts. Massage includes both light movements on the skin and deep, vigorous movements that can produce pain. Massage for pain control often includes the use of light mechanical vibrators.

Manipulation refers to a variety of twistings, pullings and stretchings, sometimes gentle, at other times quite forceful. Osteopaths and chiropractors as well as physical therapists, physiatrists and orthopedists (bone specialists) often use manipulation to treat certain types of chronic pain conditions. The results are mixed, with both failures and successes. Even when massage or manipulation is successful in relieving pain, it is still not clear why it works—exactly what the physical therapist or chiropractor is doing in the massage or manipulation technique that is responsible for the pain reduction.

It should be pointed out, however, that the California Chiropractic Association, in a number of full-page ads in magazines like *Newsweek* in 1995, cited a recent milestone study involving a multidisciplinary panel of health-care experts. In this study, the Agency for Health Care Policy and Research (AHCPR) of the U.S. Department of Health and Human Services concluded that *spinal manipulation appears to be the safest initial type of treatment for acute low-back problems in adults.* It recommended that in the majority of cases, such conservative manipulation treatment should be attempted before surgical interventions are considered.

The CCA also noted that another study conducted by the RAND Corporation concluded that spinal manipulation was an appropriate intervention for acute low-back pain. This study indicated that about 94 percent of all manipulations are performed by doctors of chiropractic or chiropractors.

Heat therapy. Heat therapy is another sensory-modulation method for pain control. Heat can be produced in a number of ways, including the use of electrically heated pads for superficial local heat and of ultrasound (pressure waves at high frequency) for deep local heat. Diathermy is a specific method for heating a limb or a part of the body from the middle outward by using electromagnetic radiation at frequencies that pass through the body (without affecting the skin) and are absorbed in the deep tissues of the body where they are transformed into heat. Heat seems to be effective particularly for low to moderate levels of pain due to deep-tissue damage such as bruises, torn muscles and ligaments, and arthritis. It is not clear why heat therapy is effective for such pain control. It seems most likely that heat therapy and other methods of physical therapy can reduce pain by producing sensory or physical inputs that eventually close the pain gates in the central nervous system, either by activating large fibers or by triggering brain processes that send inhibitory messages down to close the spinal pain gate.

Electrical stimulation of nerves, spinal cord and brain. One of the most exciting developments in the sensory control of pain since the gate-control theory was proposed in 1965 has been the use of electrical stimulation of peripheral nerves, spinal cord (e.g., dorsal column stimulation) and even brain areas (e.g., sensory thalamus) for pain relief. The most well-known and widely used of these methods has been *transcutaneous (across the skin) electrical nerve stimulation,* or TENS, based on the pioneering work of Wall and Sweet first reported in 1967.

TENS is actually a simple technique for stimulating peripheral nerves by placing electrodes on the skin surface. The electrodes today are usually made of silicone and are in contact with the skin via a conducting paste. They are connected to a battery-operated, pocket-sized stimulator capable of emitting a continuous series of electrical pulses. Different stimulators are capable of producing varying frequencies and durations of such electrical pulses, which the pain patient can control, usually by raising the level of stimulation to the point where he or she experiences a comfortable tingling. The evidence is clear now that TENS is an effective method for the treatment of chronic pain, having effects greater than a placebo machine.

The pain relief typically produced is remarkable, often outlasting the short duration of stimulation (usually 15-30 minutes) by several hours. Patients with damage to nerves or with pain in a small, localized area seem to benefit most. TENS is less effective for pain that is more widespread and less localized. Hundreds of thousands of pain patients have used TENS since the early 1970s, and many companies are now making and marketing TENS machines.

TENS machines can be obtained by medical prescription from a physician. Although this is an effective method for the sensory control of pain, it is more successful when it is used in conjunction with other pain control methods. Sternbach has noted that when used alone, TENS provides significant pain relief for about 50 percent of pain patients, dropping to 30-35 percent a year later. However, when TENS is used as part of a more comprehensive pain management program that includes other pain control methods, its success rate goes up to about 65 to 70 percent initially, maintaining around 50 percent after a year.[2]

TENS is a safe method for sensory control of pain and seems to have almost no harmful side effects. Skin irritations may occur due to the electrode paste or tape used, but nonallergic paste and nonabrasive tape are available. Some cautions regarding the proper use of TENS machines or units include *not* using them while sleeping or driving or around microwave ovens or water.[3] Patients with cardiac pacemakers may also not be able to use them, unless they have newer pacemakers that are protected against the electrical stimulation of TENS machines.

The effectiveness of TENS may be due to stimulation of large fibers that tend to close the spinal pain gate, distraction from pain by the tingling sensations, or the release of endorphins, the body's natural painkillers in the spinal cord and brain as a result of the electrical stimulation. Or the success may be due to a combination of these factors.[4] Conventional TENS involves the use of fairly mild, rapid electrical pulses that lead to a tingling or "pins-and-needles" sensation. For severe chronic pain, a more intense form of TENS with a lower pulse rate has also been used successfully, sometimes producing even greater and larger pain relief than conventional TENS.[5] Intense TENS will be discussed again later in this chapter.

Acupuncture and folk medicine. Melzack and Wall have described a number of folk medicine methods for pain control that have existed for many centuries, across different cultures, with one common characteristic: they fight pain with pain, by using brief, moderately intense pain to eliminate or reduce severe, prolonged pain.[6] One well-known example (which is also one of the oldest) is *cupping.* In this folk-medicine method a glass cup is heated and then turned upside down over the painful area of the body and pressed against it. Eventually, after some cooling causes contraction of the cup, a partial vacuum is created such that the skin gets sucked up into the cup, resulting in some skin bruising with tenderness and pain. This lesser discomfort takes the mind off the more severe pain! Cupping has been used and continues to be used for ailments like headaches, backaches and arthritic pain.

The best-known example of an ancient pain-control method that uses pain to relieve pain is *acupuncture,* which has been practiced by the Chinese for thousands of years, perhaps since as early as 3000 B.C. It involves the insertion of fine needles, usually made of steel, gold or other metals, through particular points in the skin and then twirling the needles for some time slowly. Acupuncture charts are very complex, usually with 361 points lying on 14 meridians named mostly after internal organs (e.g., large intestine, heart, bladder).

Acupuncture points are strikingly similar to *trigger points* in the body. When pressure is applied to such trigger points, it produces referred pain in nearby areas of the body. Melzack found that when intense TENS was used at trigger points or acupuncture points for severe clinical pain, the twenty-minute period of intense TENS produced pain relief for several hours, and occasionally even for days or weeks! He has therefore called acupuncture, intense TENS and other related sensory-modulation methods for pain control *hyperstimulation analgesia,* otherwise known as "counter-irritation" methods where pain is used to alleviate pain. The effectiveness of acupuncture has been shown to be due to the intense stimulation used, not so much to the precise site of the stimulation. Melzack therefore concludes that such hyperstimulation analgesic methods work because they trigger brain processes to send inhibitory messages down to close the spinal pain gate as well as other pain gates higher up in the central nervous system, leading to pain relief. Another example of hyperstimulation analgesia is *cold therapy,* usually involving the use of ice packs under a couple of layers of towels applied to the painful area for about twenty minutes, or the use of ice-block massage for about ten minutes or until numbness is experienced.

TENS, whether conventional or intense, requires a medical prescription by a physician and professional instruction and supervision. Acupuncture can be practiced only by trained and licensed acupuncture specialists. Your doctor or physician may be able to help you contact a qualified acupuncturist if you are interested in this particular form of pain treatment. You should be careful, if you are a Christian, about which acupuncturist you consult, because there are acupuncturists who use New Age thinking and methods that are incompatible with Christian faith. New Age methods such as channeling and the use of spirit guides are actually spiritually dangerous and may be demonic in origin.

Other Physical Methods for Pain Control

Exercise. Many people with chronic pain feel isolated and immobilized, spending inordinate amounts of time alone at home and in bed because of the severe, intense pain they are experiencing, whether in the lower-back region, in the face and head area or in some other part of the body. Such inactivity often worsens the pain condition, and the social isolation can lead to feelings of loneliness, boredom, frustration, depression and helplessness. *Exercise* is therefore another important physical method for pain control. It works directly by activating large fibers through appropriate movements, thus tending to close the spinal pain gate, and, if it is aerobic exercise (e.g., biking, jogging, fast walking, swimming) by stimulating an increase in brain chemicals such as serotonin and possibly enkephalin or endorphin, thus raising pain tolerance as well as having some antidepressant effects. And physical exercise also helps indirectly by strengthening muscles and joints, increasing stamina and endurance and improving general physical fitness and health.

The word *exercise* can refer to specific movements and stretches prescribed by physical therapists or physiatrists for the physical rehabilitation and recovery of damaged muscles or joints that have caused pain. Or *exercise* can refer to more general activities (e.g., walking, water exercises, using indoor exercise equipment like treadmills or stationary bikes) or weight-resistance workouts (using free weights or machines) that are done at least three times a week for thirty to forty-five minutes in order to physically condition the body. Such exercises should first be approved by a physician or physical therapist, especially for someone with a pain condition. Some types of general exercises are *not* appropriate for certain pain conditions. Exercise should also be implemented gradually and carefully.[7]

Regular exercise, whether of the specific rehabilitation type or the more general conditioning type, should be part and parcel of any pain management program. In order to live with pain effectively and to overcome chronic pain as much as possible, you would be wise to include regular exercise as part of your lifestyle, after checking with your physician first regarding what exercises would be helpful and appropriate for you. It is also possible to incorporate exercise into your schedule and lifestyle by engaging in what Dr. Bryant Stamford and Porter Shimer have described as small, nonstructured bouts of activity that are a natural part of your life, focusing on the fun of fitness without grueling exercise.[8] For example, you can walk up the stairs instead of taking the elevator or escalator in a high-rise building or shopping mall, or you can park your car further away so you can walk more. Taking "miniwalks" several times a day, for a few minutes each time, is another idea.

A unique way of exercise called Relaxercise, based on the acclaimed work of Dr. Moshe Feldenkrais, consists of a number of easy exercises that take only fifteen to thirty minutes to do. Relaxercise has apparently helped many people to feel better and obtain relief from aches and pains, with improvement in posture and flexibility as well as stress reduction.[9]

Nutrition. What you do or move, in terms of exercise, is crucial for pain control, but what you eat is also important! Chronic pain sufferers often do not eat nutritiously—or they overeat because of inactivity and boredom and therefore may end up putting on extra pounds in body weight, adding another health problem to an already painful condition. Proper nutrition is crucial for healthy living, and there are many good books available on this topic. Stamford and Shimer have some good suggestions on nutrition and weight control, or how to eat better and weigh less.[10]

Excess body weight can contribute to making a pain condition worse. Eating smaller but more frequent meals (e.g., five meals a day) coupled with regular exercise can help you lose weight, if this is necessary for you.

More specifically for people suffering from chronic pain, Sternbach strongly advocates the avoidance of stimulants or those substances which increase muscle tension and blood pressure, namely *caffeine* and *nicotine.* Caffeine is found in coffee, tea, colas, chocolate and some nonprescription painkillers, and nicotine is found in tobacco. Drinking or eating substances containing caffeine or smoking tobacco will lead to an increase in tension, irritability, nervousness and muscle tension, so that there is a higher probability that you may get a cramp or muscle spasm, which of course can worsen any pain you may already have.

Dr. Margaret Caudill, in her very helpful book *Managing Pain Before It Manages You,* makes the following suggestions for managing pain through nutrition: Do eat breakfast; don't fast for long periods or eat sweets as snacks if you suffer from hypoglycemia; don't skip meals or eat most of your calories in the evening; brief fasting and an individualized gluten-free vegetarian diet may be somewhat helpful for people with rheumatoid arthritis; low-protein and high-complex-carbohydrate diets associated with increases in serotonin may decrease pain in the central nervous system; try to avoid caffeine, alcohol, MSG and aspartame because they may worsen some pain conditions such as headaches.[11]

Sleep and rest. While inactivity can be problematic for a chronic-pain sufferer, too much activity and expenditure of energy without adequate sleep and rest can also worsen a pain condition by weakening your health. Too much exercise without adequate time for rest or recuperation—overtraining—can lead to muscle soreness and pain or even injury. It is therefore crucial for you to build in sufficient time for rest, and also adequate sleep each night (usually one or two hours more than you think you need, unless you are already sleeping too much by spending most of your nights and days in bed!). An important but often neglected component of stress management is having adequate sleep,[12] and this can also help pain control.

Finding the Right Combination
Sensory-modulation methods for pain control as described in this chapter can be helpful parts in a comprehensive approach to coping effectively with pain or managing chronic pain. However, there are also psychological and psychosocial methods for pain control that seem to work through the thought or brain processes that send descending inhibitory messages to close the appropriate pain gates, thus reducing pain. These methods will be described in the next chapter. They form a core and very important part of an effective pain-management program for people with chronic pain.

Roy needed to find such a program. After a sports injury during a football game, he had recurrent low-back pain over a two-year period. He tried pain medications and saw a chiropractor, but had only partial relief of his pain. He eventually tried TENS with his physician's prescription and supervision, and this sensory-modulation method for pain control helped him to experience further pain relief—but not completely.

Instead of opting for back surgery, Roy consulted a psychologist who had special experience in pain management. He learned a number of psychological and psychosocial methods for pain control that he has been using with some success. He is now able to live a fairly normal life and function almost as efficiently at work as he used to, although he still experiences some low-back pain periodically. He no longer takes pain medications; he uses the TENS machine occasionally when he needs temporary pain relief.

Roy has found that the active self-control methods for pain management which he learned from the psychologist are sufficient, most of the time, to enable him to live and cope effectively with his recurrent low-back pain. It does not occur as often; when it does, it does not affect him as badly. Roy feels that every pain patient or person suffering from a chronic-pain condition should learn such methods of pain control. They are described in the next chapter. They are not magic or panaceas, but they will help you experience some sense of control over your pain condition, even though it may still persist to some degree.

5

Psychological & Psychosocial Methods for Pain Control

J ANE HAS BEEN SUFFERING FROM CHRONIC PAIN FOR OVER TWO years. She has tension headaches almost daily, with really intense headaches about once a week. They usually last a few hours each time. She has been taking pain medications but with only limited relief. The headaches have generally persisted in frequency and intensity despite the pills, and she has recently decided to stop taking more pain medications because she is afraid of becoming overdependent on them.

Jane works long hours as an accounts clerk in a downtown business company that had to reduce staff a couple of years ago as a cost-cutting strategy necessitated by the economic recession. Her work hours had to be increased from eight hours a day to ten to twelve hours a day. Her job has therefore become much more demanding and stressful. To make things worse, she also has a boss who has become increasingly impatient and cranky. He has set unrealistic work loads and deadlines for the office staff, several of whom have resigned because they could not continue to work under such conditions. Jane needs her job desperately and is not confident that she can get another job that pays as well, so she has hung in there. However, she has been experiencing tension headaches almost daily.

Out of desperation and frustration, Jane recently decided to consult a clinical psychologist who is experienced in treating pain patients. She has been seeing the psychologist for the past two months and has learned a number of psychological techniques for pain control that have helped her to cope more effectively with her headaches. She still has daily headaches, but they are not as intense and do not last as long. She is glad that she consulted the psychologist and feels hopeful that she will be able to cope with her headache pain without medications from now on. Since her headaches appear to be stress-related, she has found the stress-management strategies covered in her sessions with the psychologist helpful for both stress and pain control.

This chapter will describe the major psychological and psychosocial methods that have been developed, with some success, for use by people suffering from pain conditions. These options for pain control may help you, like Jane, to manage chronic pain more effectively.

Chronic pain often is still present, no matter what we do. But, overall, many pain patients have found the following techniques helpful for reducing their suffering and sometimes even their level of pain. Most of these techniques are cognitive-behavioral ones—they have to do with helping you change the way you *think* (cognitive) and the way you *act* or *behave* (behavioral) in order to change your feelings or experiences, including the reduction of negative experiences like anxiety, depression and chronic pain.[1]

Relaxation Techniques
Certain chronic pain conditions, such as tension headaches and even low-back pain, can be worsened by tension, both physical and mental. Hence, techniques that help you to relax away muscle or physical tension as well as calm you down mentally can help you control your pain as well. There are many different versions of relaxation tech-

niques available today. Let me suggest and describe just a couple of them: (1) progressive muscle relaxation and (2) a stress-management or stress-inoculation approach that includes slow, deep breathing, calming self-talk and pleasant imagery.

1. Progressive Muscle Relaxation. This relaxation technique involves the alternate tensing and then relaxing or letting go of various muscle parts of your body. Again there are several variations of progressive muscle relaxation involving various muscle parts and major muscle groups. The following are the instructions for trying progressive muscle relaxation using four major muscle groups.

First sit in a comfortable chair or recliner, in a room and at a time when you will not be disturbed. Give yourself at least 15-20 minutes of uninterrupted "relaxation time" to practice the relaxation exercises, beginning with the leg muscles and ending with the arm muscles.

Leg muscles. You can tense your thigh and calf muscles by pointing your toes toward your face and tensing these muscles hard. Hold the tension for 7-10 seconds by counting slowly up to 5. Then let go and allow the muscles to go limp. Now use self-talk: tell yourself to "just relax, let go of all the tension . . . allow the muscles to smooth out . . . take it easy . . . just unwind and relax more and more . . ." Continue with this relaxation patter for 20 seconds or so before proceeding to repeat this exercise. Do this exercise a total of 4 times. Then proceed to the next one.

Upper-body muscles. After completing the exercise for the leg muscles, focus your attention on the muscles of your upper body—your chest, stomach, shoulders and back. Tense them by taking in a slow, deep breath, holding it for a count up to 5 (about 7-10 seconds), pulling your stomach in, and arching your back. When you reach a count of 5, slowly exhale and let go of all the muscle tension, again telling yourself mentally to relax and take it easy, using the relaxation patter or self-talk for about 20 seconds or so before repeating the exercise. Do it a total of 4 times.

Some authors emphasize that you should inhale using *diaphragmatic breathing*: with each breath you take in, your abdomen expands and not your chest. *Chest breathing* refers to your chest expanding (and not your abdomen) with each breath you take in. Diaphragmatic breathing is supposedly better, and if you can train yourself to breathe in this way, fine. However, if you are more comfortable using chest breathing, this is okay too, as long as you practice breathing in slowly and exhaling the tension slowly. Do not engage in shallow, quick breathing, which is hyperventilation!

If, in doing any of these relaxation exercises, you feel dizzy or uncomfortable or experience pain, you should stop. For example, some pain conditions, such as severe back pain, may not allow you to arch your back. Dr. Caudill has pointed out that for some pain patients who also have seizure disorders, insulin-dependent diabetes or hypertension (high blood pressure), relaxation techniques may have some inadvertent negative effects initially, so they should be used with some caution and modification. For example, if you also have a seizure disorder, it may be safer for you to start practicing relaxation techniques while lying down, in case you trigger a seizure. But relaxation techniques can often help seizure patients to eventually control their seizures better. Diabetic patients may experience hypoglycemic reactions due to relaxation, and may therefore need to reduce their insulin intake if necessary after consultation with their physicians. Those with hypertension or high blood pressure should slowly change postural positions (for example, from sitting to standing). After mastering relaxation techniques that may lead to reductions in blood pressure, they should check with their physicians to see if they can have their antihypertensive medications reduced.[2]

After doing this exercise for the upper-body muscles 4 times, you are ready to proceed to the next exercise.

Face and neck muscles. Focus your attention now on the muscles of your face and neck regions. Tense these muscles by closing your eyes tightly, biting your teeth (*not* your tongue!), smiling back, pushing your chin down as if to touch your chest but not allowing it to touch your chest. Hold the tension for a count up to 5 (7-10 seconds), and then relax and let go of these muscles, again using the relaxation patter or self-talk for up to 20 seconds or so. Repeat this exercise for a total of 4 times before proceeding to the final exercise.

Arm muscles. Now focus your attention on the muscles of your arms. Tense them by clenching your fists and flexing your biceps (as if you are posing in a body-building contest!). Hold the tension for a count up to 5 (7-10 seconds), and then relax and let your arms flop down limp by your sides. Again, engage in the relaxation patter or self-talk for 20 seconds or so before repeating the exercise, doing it a total of 4 times.

By the time you have finished doing all 4 exercises (for the 4 major muscle groups) a total of 4 times for each of them, you will have completed 16 exercises (4 times 4 exercises). At the end you should give yourself a couple more minutes to just sit quietly and enjoy the feelings of deeper and more complete muscle relaxation that you are experiencing by this time. Then, count from 1 to 5 as you slowly move your muscles, and eventually open your eyes at the count of 5, feeling very relaxed and refreshed. This version of progressive-muscle-relaxation technique should take about 15 minutes or so and should be practiced once daily, perhaps just before bedtime, but earlier if you tend to fall asleep before completing the relaxation exercises! They should not be practiced immediately after a meal.

Many pain patients have found it helpful to practice progressive-muscle-relaxation exercises daily until they have mastered the ability to relax deeply and quickly even without going through all the exercises. They are then able to relax quickly just by taking in a few slow, deep breaths whenever they feel tense or experience the beginning of some pain, for example, a mild headache coming on. Some pain patients have been able to relax away the tension so well that the tension headache does not materialize fully, and therefore they are able to control their headache pain effectively. It may also be helpful for you to use a "reminder trigger" (such as when you look at your watch or pick up the phone) to remind yourself to do a few brief relaxation exercises—for example, taking a few slow, deep breaths and telling yourself to "just relax."

2. Stress Management/Inoculation Relaxation Techniques. In a stress management or stress-inoculation approach to relaxation, especially as developed by Dr. Donald Meichenbaum and his colleagues,[3] three major relaxation techniques are used.

Slow, deep breathing. This is similar to the second exercise for the upper-body muscles just described for progressive muscle relaxation, but using only the slow, deep breathing. Again inhale slowly, hold your breath for a few seconds, noticing the tension rising, and then exhale the tension out slowly. Diaphragmatic breathing is preferred, but chest breathing is okay too. You can repeat this exercise a few times and then go back to normal breathing.

Calming self-talk. This second technique is similar to the relaxation patter or self-talk described earlier. You can say a number of calming statements to yourself, for example, "Just relax, take it easy, let go of all the tension, allow the muscles to smooth out . . ."

Pleasant imagery. This third and final technique involves the use of your imagination to visualize a pleasant, enjoyable and relaxing scene, for example, lying on the beach in Hawaii, taking a walk in the woods, watching a beautiful sunset or sunrise, or a majestic mountain and waterfall. Everyone has his or her own favorite pleasant and relaxing scenes or mental pictures. Use whatever helps you to relax even more deeply and comfortably. Many Christians prefer to use biblical imagery such as Psalm 23—they picture themselves lying down in green pastures, right beside quiet or still waters, resting in the Lord as their Shepherd. The use of such pleasant imagery can be very helpful if you are able to image such scenes easily. Some people have difficulty imaging, and for them progressive-muscle-relaxation exercises or some other type of relaxation technique may be more effective. The use of pleasant imagery for the Christian consists simply of making use of the imaginative powers given us by our Creator. It does *not* include other imagery techniques, often used by New Age authors, that involve contacting an "inner guide" who basically functions as a "familiar spirit." Such New Age imagery and meditative techniques are often related to the occult and are demonic in nature.

Another well-known relaxation technique is a passive, quiet meditative exercise developed and described by Dr. Herbert Benson to bring about what he has called the "relaxation response."[4] It basically involves sitting quietly in a comfortable position with your eyes closed; deeply relaxing all your muscles from your feet up to your face; breathing through your nose and saying a word like *one* whenever you breathe out, for a total of about 20 minutes; and maintaining a quiet and passive attitude throughout, even if distracting thoughts occur. Some Christians may have trouble with this meditative relaxation technique because it is too similar to Transcendental Meditation, or TM. However, it does *not* use mantras per se, and the quieting down may be helpful to some people who tend to rush around a lot and have many racing thoughts. A Christian approach to meditation will be described in more detail in a later chapter of this book. TM and other Eastern or New Age meditative techniques, especially those employing mantras, which are names of Hindu deities, should of course not be used by Christians, because of the spiritual risk involved and the possibility of demonic attack.

Cognitive Coping Skills

In addition to relaxation techniques, there are several other *cognitive coping skills* that some pain patients have found useful for pain control. They include the following techniques.[5]

Imaginative inattention: ignoring the pain by using imagery or visualization that is incompatible with the experience of pain. This is really a *distraction strategy*, examples of which include imagining yourself enjoying a pleasant day at the beach, in the country or at a social event.

Imaginative transformation of pain: acknowledging the noxious or unpleasant sensations but interpreting them as something other than pain, or minimizing them as unreal or trivial. For example, instead of focusing on your sports-related knee pain as pain, you reinterpret and transform it into "tightness" or "numbness" but *not* pain.

Imaginative transformation of context: acknowledging the noxious or unpleasant sensations but transforming or reinterpreting their context or setting. For example, if you have arthritic pain in your elbow or wrist, you imagine or picture yourself instead as James Bond, having been shot in the elbow or wrist, driving a car down a winding mountain road while being chased by enemy agents, but you succeed in your mission in preventing the outbreak of World War III. Children with pain, in particular, may find this technique helpful.

Attention-diversion (external): focusing attention on physical characteristics of the environment rather than on the pain itself. This is another distraction strategy. For example, instead of focusing on your toothache or headache while attending a class, you start counting ceiling tiles or observe articles of clothing of the people around you.

Attention-diversion (internal): focusing attention on self-generated, internal thoughts that are non-imagery-produced. Again this is a distraction strategy. For example, instead of focusing on your headache pain, you start doing mental arithmetic or making a list of words of popular songs.

Somatization: focusing on the part of your body experiencing the noxious or intense sensations but in a detached manner. For example, you do pay attention to the low-back pain you are experiencing, but you act as if you are a scientist writing a biology report on the sensations you are experiencing in your low-back area, so that you analyze them in a detached, scientific, experimental way. *Somatization* is simply the label that has been used for this strategy of focused "detachment"; it should not be confused with the more technical term of the same name that refers to the expression of emotional distress in physical or somatic symptoms.

These cognitive coping skills do not always work for everyone suffering from different pain conditions. But they can be useful for providing you with some sense of control over your pain experiences by giving you several options or techniques you can use to cope more effectively with your pain. Several of these techniques involve distraction from your pain and paying attention to other more pleasant thoughts or images.

However, some of these techniques actually involve *attending* to the painful experiences but in ways that help you to cope better. Dr. Jon Kabat-Zinn, founder and director of the Stress Reduction Clinic at the University of Massachusetts Medical Center, has actually instructed patients with pain conditions to remember that they are trying to find out about their pain, to learn from it, to know it better, and not to stop it or get rid of it or escape from it. He has used relaxation and *mindful-meditation* techniques that focus on one's breathing in and out repeatedly and quietly in a sitting position, as well as other strategies. One is the *body scan* technique of breathing in and out while focusing on one part of the body at a time (for example, the toes) until the whole body from toes to head has been scanned or focused on in a deliberate, mindful way. Another strategy is *yoga exercises.* He reports having good results with such stress and pain-management techniques with patients experiencing various kinds of chronic-pain conditions.[6]

While Christians will not be interested in using certain types of meditation and yoga techniques rooted in Buddhism or New Age thinking, because they are spiritually risky or dangerous, learning to focus on your pain in quiet and prayerful ways (ways that are part and parcel of Christian meditation) can be helpful, especially if the distraction strategies do not work for you. Christian meditation and other spiritual resources for living with pain more effectively will be covered later in this book.

Cognitive Therapy Methods

Cognitive therapy is an approach to psychotherapy or counseling that basically helps people deal with their problem feelings such as anxiety, depression, anger, even pain experiences, by changing their basic assumptions and self-talk—in other words, their thinking or cognitions. Dr. Aaron Beck is the founder of Cognitive Therapy and Dr. Albert Ellis originated Rational-Emotive Therapy, the two leading schools of Cognitive Therapy. Another well-known approach called Cognitive-Behavior Modification has been associated mainly with Meichenbaum's work. Several Christian approaches to Cognitive Therapy have also been developed in recent years, with Misbelief Therapy originated by Dr. William Backus probably being the best known.[7]

Basically, cognitive therapy methods for pain control focus on helping you identify and then change maladaptive, unhelpful, negative, unreasonable, unrealistic and extreme ways of thinking that often underlie emotional problems—and that can also worsen your pain experience, since anxiety, tension and depression can add to your suffering from pain. Such unbiblical ways of thinking have been labeled as *misbeliefs* by Dr. Backus. After identifying the misbeliefs, you need to tell yourself the truth and replace the misbeliefs with more accurate, biblical, realistic, balanced and reasonable ways of thinking that can help you feel less anxious, depressed, tense or angry, or that can even cause you to experience less pain.

Without going into too many details, here are some cognitive therapy methods that can help you cope more effectively with pain:

Using an A-B-C diary. An A-B-C diary is simply a form of daily journal in which you write your thoughts and feelings, including experiences of pain. *A* stands for Activating events or situations that trigger negative emotional experiences or behavioral responses. Such experiences or responses are recorded under *C,* or Consequences (emotional and/or behavioral). *B* is the key—it stands for your Beliefs or misbeliefs, referring to the negative, extreme, unrealistic, irrational, unbiblical self-talk that often is at the root of negative emotional experiences. In other words, A does not lead to C directly but triggers B—and it is your thinking *(B)* usually that contributes to your eventual feelings *(C)*.

For example, let's say you have had a bad day at work because of a cranky boss who was very critical and impatient with you. You arrive home feeling angry, anxious and somewhat depressed. You also have a splitting headache, which is not unfamiliar to you because you suffer from frequent tension headaches, often on a daily basis. In using the A-B-C diary, you might make the following notes:

A	B	C
Bad day at work, cranky boss.	I can't take this anymore. I can't handle the stress at work. I feel weak, and my headaches are getting worse. Oh, the pain—my head is bursting! This is too much for me!	Angry, anxious, a bit depressed. A splitting headache.

You realize from the self-talk or thoughts recorded under *B* that you are saying negative things to yourself that are probably making you feel worse emotionally as well as intensifying your headache pain. The next step you need to take is to challenge your negative self-talk or misbeliefs.

Challenging and changing misbeliefs. It may be helpful for you to begin by asking the following questions about your thoughts, misbeliefs or self-talk: *On what basis do I say this? Where is the evidence for my negative conclusions? Is there another way of thinking about this situation? So what if it's true that I am weak and not doing that well at work—what does this mean to me? What does God have to say about this in the Bible?*

These questions can help you to think things through so that you come to more accurate, biblical, balanced and reasonable conclusions. For example, you may end up saying the following (more biblical) coping self-talk: *It's been a bad day and I didn't cope so well. But my boss was really cranky and difficult; it's not all my fault. Besides, I survived! We all have good and bad days. I know I'm having a splitting headache and my head feels like it's going to burst. But with God's help, I can calm down, pray, do my relaxation exercises and just let go of the tension. I can cope with this headache—it's not the end of the world. I'll be okay soon.*

Certain *common patterns of distorted thinking* have been well described by Dr. David Burns in his book *Feeling Good.*[8] They include *all-or-nothing thinking* (seeing things in extremes with no middle ground), *overgeneralization* (taking one negative incident and assuming it holds true for all places and at all times), *mental filter,* or selective attention to only the negatives, *disqualifying the positive, jumping to conclusions* (with little or no evidence at all), *catastrophizing,* or magnifying the bad, *emotional reasoning* (if you *feel* it, then it must be true), *personalization* (blaming yourself even if it was not all your fault) and so forth. Such thinking needs to be identified, challenged and eventually replaced with more accurate, balanced and biblical thinking.

Christians in particular may have some unbiblical beliefs or misbeliefs, such as the following ones noted by Dr. Chris Thurman, with Scriptures that challenge them:

"Because I'm a good Christian, God will protect me from pain and suffering" (see Jn 16:33; Phil 1:29; 1 Pet 4:12-13).

"A good Christian doesn't feel angry, anxious or depressed" (see Mk 11:15-16; Mk 14:32-34; Jn 11:33-35; Eph 4:26).[9]

Challenging and changing misbeliefs and patterns of distorted thinking can help you put things in perspective and see things from God's viewpoint, so that you end up coping better and living more effectively with your pain condition.

Stress-Inoculation Training

Stress-inoculation training refers to a more comprehensive cognitive-behavioral approach to the management not only of pain but also of anxiety and anger.[10] Originally developed by Meichenbaum and his colleagues, it consists of three main phases.

The first phase for pain control is an *educational phase* in which you are provided a rationale or conceptual framework for understanding pain experience and pain management. The Melzack-Wall gate-control theory already described is the one usually used.

The second phase is a *rehearsal* or *acquisition phase* in which you are exposed to a variety of cognitive and behavioral techniques for pain control, such as the ones already covered in this chapter. You are allowed, however, to choose the ones you prefer, according to your individual needs and experiences so far. You then rehearse or practice each of these pain-control techniques briefly, with the therapist modeling for you and "coaching" or guiding you. The most commonly chosen techniques for pain control, in this second phase, include relaxation and slow, deep breathing; distraction; imagery techniques; and coping or calming self-talk.

The third and final phase of stress-inoculation training is an *application phase* in which you have the opportunity to apply or test out your newly acquired pain-control skills in a number of possible ways. For example, you might try imagery rehearsal in which you imagine yourself having a pain experience such as a bad headache or low-back-pain episode and then using the techniques to reduce the tension and pain. Another way is to do role-playing with your therapist in which you reverse roles: you play the role of the therapist guiding and training the pain patient (played by the therapist) in the cognitive and behavioral skills for pain control.

One more way to approach the application phase is exposure to an actual experimental pain stressor, such as immersing your hand in ice-cold water, eventually leading to some pain experience in your hand. Throughout the task, however, you will be applying the pain-control skills you have learned so as to increase your pain tolerance during this task.

Stress-inoculation training can also be used to *prepare* yourself for an upcoming acute pain situation, such as having dental work done, as well as to cope with the acute pain during such a procedure. It can therefore be applied to both acute and chronic pain situations.

Prepared-Childbirth Training

Another example of a basically psychological method for pain management is *prepared-childbirth training*, in which pregnant women are taught a number of coping skills such as relaxation, special breathing techniques, and attention-focusing on a spot on the wall or ceiling, to be used during the childbirth process to control or reduce pain.

Prepared-childbirth training may help some women to experience less childbirth pain, but it does not necessarily eliminate such pain. Melzack and Wall have pointed out that the average pain reduction reported as a result of prepared-childbirth training is relatively small, though statistically significant.[11] There is a need, therefore, for further refinement of these obviously helpful techniques for pain control.

Biofeedback

Biofeedback refers to the use of sensitive electronic equipment to monitor and provide feedback on a person's brain waves or EEG, blood pressure, heart rate or muscle tension in order to help him or her to achieve voluntary control over such biological processes. For certain chronic-pain conditions, biofeedback has been used to help pain patients learn to relax and reduce muscle tension in order to control tension headache or back pain, or to change their brain waves to the "alpha" pattern (steady 8-12 cycles per second) associated with relaxed meditative states in order to reduce pain.

Melzack and Wall conclude that the research shows that relaxation training alone is usually as effective as biofeedback training for tension and migraine headaches, low-back pain and other chronic-pain conditions. However, biofeedback *does* contribute significantly to psychological treatment for pain. It seems to enhance psychological pain control by acting as a useful means for distraction of attention, suggestion, relaxation and a sense of control over pain.[12] If you are interested in obtaining biofeedback training to help you with your pain management, you can ask your physician for a referral to a qualified biofeedback therapist or to a pain clinic which offers biofeedback training.

Hypnosis

Hypnosis usually involves instructions and suggestions from a qualified hypnotherapist to help facilitate the occurrence of a trance state in the person with chronic pain such that pain is reduced or eliminated. After reviewing the research on the effectiveness of hypnosis for clinical pain control, Melzack and Wall noted that there was still virtually no reliable evidence from well-controlled clinical studies to show that hypnosis was more effective than a placebo pill or simple encouragement and moral support from the family physician or clergy. They therefore concluded that hypnosis by itself could not be considered a reliably useful therapy for clinical pain.[13]

However, more recent research from controlled clinical studies has shown hypnosis to be as effective as or more effective than other types of psychological interventions for pain control.[14]

Some Christians have serious reservations, if not objections, to hypnosis as a psychological method of therapy or pain reduction. It is beyond the scope of this book to discuss further the issues involved in the use of hypnosis from a Christian perspective. Suffice it to say that hypnosis should always be approached with great caution.

Operant Conditioning or Reinforcement

Operant-conditioning or reinforcement methods for pain control, based on the views of Dr. B. F. Skinner, have been advocated and applied primarily by Dr. Wilbert E. Fordyce, a behavioral psychologist who has worked with chronic-pain patients especially in inpatient treatment programs. Operant-conditioning methods basically use rewards for well behavior and penalties or punishments for pain behavior, viewing pain mainly as a behavior (i.e., verbal complaints of pain) that has been reinforced or rewarded by people such as family members, friends and physicians around the pain patient.

Dr. Fordyce's strict inpatient operant conditioning or retraining program for patients who are suffering from chronic pain requires them to be hospitalized for an average of eight weeks, during which all their usual "crutches" are taken away. All pain behaviors or complaints are ignored, whereas all physical movements or "well behaviors" are rewarded with praise or smiles. Pain medication is gradually reduced to the bare minimum, a process called "detoxification." Fordyce has found that his patients end up becoming more active, complaining less of pain, taking fewer pain medications, working more and generally leading more normal lives.

Melzack and Wall have noted limitations and problems with Fordyce's approach, including the need to deal more directly with a patient's subjective experience of pain and not just the external pain behaviors or complaints. Also such an inpatient program is very costly. Further, there is a need for better-controlled clinical studies or evaluations of this inpatient treatment, especially using "attention-placebo" control groups that control for the simple effects of giving attention and support to pain patients.[15]

Yet conditioning is significant. It may be helpful for you to reflect on whether your pain experience may be a behavior that has been rewarded with increased attention from people around you and relief from certain unpleasant responsibilities. It may be helpful for you to deliberately schedule rewards to yourself or from your loved ones when you engage in *well* behaviors rather than complaints of pain.

Pacing and Pleasurable Activities

Sternbach has recommended *pacing activities* as another important psychological method for chronic pain control.[16] In order to manage your pain more effectively, you need to pace the activities of your day in such a way that you do a task only as long as you do *not* experience a significant increase in pain. In other words, you should stop an activity just *before* your pain gets worse, switching to some more pleasant activity or taking a relaxation break. Pacing yourself and your activities in this way can help you to get the most out of each day, without experiencing significantly more pain.

In addition to pacing wisely, you may also find it helpful to schedule into your day more *pleasurable activities* that you enjoy doing, without straining yourself or overdoing it. For example, you may find it helpful to listen to your favorite music more often, to spend more time reading books you enjoy or to treat yourself more often to a nice long bath. Some people suffering from chronic pain refrain from pleasurable activities that they enjoy doing because they allow their pain to control them too much. For example, a pain patient may not play golf, though he or she enjoys it very much, because of headaches. Such a person can still enjoy playing golf, to a certain extent, *despite* the headaches. In fact, playing golf with friends may actually help this pain patient to suffer less from the headaches—concentrating more on pleasant social interaction and the pleasure of playing golf can be a good distraction from pain.

If you suffer from a chronic-pain condition, make sure you have your physician's approval before doing any strenuous physical activity. Then, schedule more of such pleasant events or activities into your daily or weekly program with appropriate pacing so that you can still enjoy life to a certain extent and live more effectively with your pain.

Psychotherapy

Some people who have chronic pain also have other psychological or psychiatric problems: significant struggles with depression, anxiety, anger, stress, marital and family difficulties. If you are experiencing such problems to a significant extent and for a long enough period of time so that you feel you can't go on without some extra help, you may find it helpful to consult a professional therapist for counseling or psychotherapy. The therapist may be a licensed psychologist, psychiatrist, clinical social worker, marriage and family therapist, professional counselor, pastoral counselor or psychiatric nurse. Your physician may be able to refer you to a good licensed therapist. If there are serious marital or family problems, you may particularly want to consult someone specially trained or experienced in marital and family therapy. Some professional therapists not only can help with your psychological or emotional struggles but also can provide you with pain-control interventions such as those described in this book.

Christian patients or clients often prefer to seek professional therapists who are Christians. If you are having trouble finding a Christian therapist, you may want to contact the following Christian organizations for names and addresses of Christian therapists in your geographical area:

Christian Association for Psychological Studies
P.O. Box 310400
New Braunfels, TX 78131-0400
(210) 629-CAPS

Focus on the Family Counseling Dept.
8605 Explorer Drive
Colorado Springs, CO 80920
(719) 531-3400

Please note that these organizations do not guarantee the quality of the professional services the counselors on their lists may provide; they act simply as referral sources. You'll need to contact a specific therapist and find out more information from him or her before deciding whether to explore professional counseling with that person.

Multiple-Convergent Therapy

Multiple-convergent therapy is a term used by Melzack and Wall to refer to pain-control interventions that combine a number of different psychological and psychosocial methods for pain management.[17] One example is a treatment that combines stress inoculation training with biofeedback training. Another example is combining relaxation, cognitive coping skills, cognitive therapy methods, and marital and family therapy. For some complex chronic-pain conditions, multifaceted treatments or multiple-convergent therapy may be needed and may be more effective than a single pain-treatment approach. In fact, Melzack and Wall conclude that multiple-convergent therapy is becoming more and more the standard psychological approach to pain control. They noted that this approach can also refer to the combination of psychological methods for pain management with pain medications or other physical, sensory-modulation procedures for pain control.[18]

Support Groups

Support groups as a type of psychosocial intervention for different kinds of problems, whether psychological or physical, have sprung up all over the country. There are support groups for people with cancer, epilepsy, arthritis, alcoholism, drug addictions, dysfunctional family backgrounds and so on. People suffering from chronic-pain conditions can benefit from forming or attending support groups for those suffering from similar conditions. Some of the support groups for cancer or arthritis patients provide opportunities for such patients to share about their pain problems and how they are attempting to cope with pain effectively in their lives. You may benefit from participating in a support group with people who have pain conditions similar to yours. Your physician may be able to provide you with further information about support groups.

This chapter has provided descriptions of the major psychological and psychosocial methods available for pain control. They have been found by at least some patients to be helpful for pain management and reduction. Cognitive-behavioral therapy in particular has been found to be effective for chronic-pain control.[19] Multiple-convergent therapy, however, appears to be most promising, as different types of pain treatments are combined for different pain patients.

Jane found several of the psychological techniques described in this chapter very helpful in the control of her headache pain. You too may find some of these methods effective for better management of your pain.

6

Pain Clinics
& Hospices

W HILE SIGNIFICANT ADVANCES HAVE BEEN MADE IN PAIN MANAGE-
ent and effective methods for pain control have been developed in recent years, the challenge of pain remains. A number of chronic-pain conditions have not yet responded well enough
to the pain treatments we have available today. Many millions of low-
back pain, migraine and tension-headache sufferers still struggle with
their chronic-pain conditions, despite the best efforts at treating their
pain. Patients suffering from the advanced or terminal stages of certain types of cancer may experience the most frightening and excruciating of all pains. Melzack and Wall point out that the *pain clinic* and
the *hospice* have been two relatively recent crucial developments in
pain treatment that have come about in response to the challenge of
the chronic-pain patient whose pain continues to persist. I will briefly
summarize their descriptions of these important innovations in pain
treatment.[1]

The Pain Clinic
A pain clinic is a place where health specialists interested specifically
in the treatment of pain can work collaboratively as a team to help

a patient with a particularly challenging, complex and chronic pain condition. The concept can be attributed to the work and experience of Dr. John J. Bonica of the University of Washington Medical School. He is a leading authority on pain treatment and an anesthesiologist by training and profession. He was not pleased with how chronic-pain patients with difficult-to-treat pain conditions arrived to see him only at the end of the line, so to speak, after having seen many other "pain doctors" (physicians specializing in pain treatment). He therefore brought together a group of specialists such as neurosurgeons, ortho-pedic surgeons, neurologists, psychiatrists, psychologists and others who were all interested in pain management. He formed a team of pain doctors and other health-care professionals, and they offered their services in the form of a pain clinic.

Pain clinics have mushroomed all over North America, and at least one can be found in each major city of the Western world. The better ones are usually, though not necessarily, associated with well-known universities, university hospitals or general hospitals. There are also several good pain clinics that are more free-standing. A list of them can be found in Sternbach's book *Mastering Pain.*[2]

There are also some so-called "pain clinics" that are nothing more than misleading relabelings of traditional pain-treatment services of-fered by one specialist, instead of by a truly multidisciplinary team of pain doctors or specialists, such as is available in a proper pain clinic. Three psychologists who have made significant contributions to pain control and research through the collaborative teamwork of pain clin-ics are Wilbert Fordyce, Richard Sternbach and Ronald Melzack (whose publications have already been cited earlier in this book).

A recent review of several representative multidisciplinary pain-treatment programs that make much use of behavioral-treatment methods included those located at the University of Washington School of Medicine; the University of California-San Diego, Veterans Administration Hospital; the Casa Colina Hospital; the Portland Pain Center; the Mayo Clinic; the Miller-Duran Hospital; and the Duke

University Medical Center.[3] These programs, usually housed in pain clinics or centers, include team members from disciplines such as nursing, physical therapy, occupational therapy, psychology, psychiatry, anesthesiology, neurosurgery and orthopedics.

Other well-known pain clinics or treatment programs include those at the Scripps Clinic and Research Foundation in La Jolla, California, where Sternbach has served as director of the Pain Treatment Center; the Department of Veterans Affairs Medical Center in Long Beach, California, where Kenneth Gerber is director of the Chronic-Pain Management Program; the Deaconess Hospital in Boston, where Margaret Caudill is codirector of the Arnold Pain Center; the Department of Anesthesiology at the University of Virginia Medical Center in Charlottesville, Virginia, where Ellen Catalano worked as a biofeedback therapist in the Pain Management Center; and the Montreal General Hospital, a McGill University teaching hospital where Melzack is director of research at the Pain Center in Montreal, Quebec, Canada. There are other good pain clinics that I have not mentioned because of space limitations.

A typical pain clinic has a single doctor or physician who is responsible for the overall coordinated treatment and follow-up of the chronic-pain patient. The patient's first visit to the clinic will be with this doctor, who will take a history of the pain condition, conduct a medical examination and order whatever tests may be necessary. This doctor can be from any of the traditional medical specialties such as anesthesiology, neurology, neurosurgery or orthopedics, but he or she has a special interest and experience in pain treatment. The doctor will then present the findings obtained on the new chronic-pain patient to the team of other specialists who work together at the pain clinic. The treatment plan emerges from their consultations and discussions together.

The pain-clinic team allows specialists or professionals from different health-related fields, including psychology and psychiatry, to learn from one another. Innovative clinical and research ideas may result from their meetings together. There are times when more basic research scientists and experimental or physiological psychologists also get involved in the pain clinic for research purposes. New pain treatments may therefore be developed and tested in a pain clinic for the benefit of both current chronic-pain patients and future ones. Data and complete patient files can be collected over a long enough period of time from large enough samples of patients so that the effectiveness of particular pain treatments can be better determined.

You may want to consult a pain clinic if there is a good one in the area or city where you live, especially if you have had a chronic-pain condition for years and traditional treatments by single-pain doctors or specialists have not helped much. Your own physician may be able to refer you to a good pain clinic, or else you may try contacting a reputable medical school or hospital in your area.

The Hospice

The hospice was developed as a special response to the challenge of the terminally ill—the dying patient, usually with advanced cancer. Melzack and Wall noted that approximately 700,000 new cases of cancer are diagnosed annually in the United States, and about 400,000 people die from cancer each year. Bonica has estimated that about 40 percent of cancer patients with intermediate stages of the disease and 60 to 80 percent of patients with advanced cancer experience moderate to severe pain.[4] In other words, most terminally ill patients with advanced cancer struggle with great pain.

Dr. Cicely Saunders is the key person in the revolution that has taken place in the treatment of dying patients, especially those with advanced cancer and severe pain. A medical doctor herself, as well as a former nurse and social worker, Dr. Saunders founded the first hospice—called St. Christopher's Hospice—in London in 1967. She and her staff of doctors, nurses and social workers, all of them seriously committed Christians, have led the way in deeply and compassionately caring for dying patients who have access to the staff around the clock. The hospice has an atmosphere of intensive caring, with no terminally ill patient left alone except by his or her own choice. Most patients live in open wards with others rather than in isolation. A few have single rooms when necessary or for personal reasons. Patients also learn to care for one another; they are enabled by the hospice environment and staff to die with dignity. The average patient at the hospice usually passes away after about twelve days, but some die sooner, and others survive for longer periods.

Patients are carefully selected to enter the hospice based on two initial strict guidelines. First, they need to be living within a particular geographical area around the hospice. Family members, relatives and friends close by can therefore visit the patients more easily. Also, they all have had some contact with or exposure to the hospice already. A hospice committee consisting of nurses, doctors and others makes the final decision, after weighing all the facts and needs of the patient, as to whether he or she should (1) be admitted to the hospice, (2) be sent elsewhere or (3) remain at home.

Saunders has also pioneered the use of narcotic drugs, including heroin and morphine, for control of the severe pain that many patients with advanced cancer experience. A combination called the Brompton Mixture, consisting of morphine, cocaine, ethyl alcohol, flavoring syrup and chloroform water, has become widely known and used for pain control of such patients. However, Melzack and Wall point out that more recent research indicates that a simpler and less costly mixture of morphine in water (with a little bit of alcohol as an antifungal and antibacterial agent) is as effective as the Brompton Mixture and is now being used to treat terminally ill patients who have severe pain. Morphine has also been found to be as effective as heroin in equivalent doses, so heroin is no longer used as often by the team at St. Christopher's Hospice.

Neither the Brompton Mixture nor the simpler morphine solution works for every patient with advanced cancer pain. Other pain-control methods are often necessary.

More recently, hospice care has also been made available to AIDS patients. However, the need is still great for better care of terminally ill AIDS patients. From a Christian ethical perspective, the provision of high-quality compassionate and humane care for terminally ill patients suffering terribly from medical conditions such as cancer or AIDS is crucial. But it should *not* include so-called "death with dignity" interventions, for example, physician-assisted suicide or other forms of lethal treatment.

The hospice is a very humane and compassionate response to the challenge of the dying patient, originally motivated by Christian love on the part of Saunders and her staff. However, it is an expensive undertaking.

An alternative to the hospice, less costly but still aimed at providing intensive caring for the terminally ill patient, was developed by Dr. Balfour Mount at the Royal Victoria Hospital in Montreal, a McGill University teaching hospital. He called it the *Palliative Care Unit (PCU)*. A PCU is a specialized ward of 10-12 beds in a large general hospital, set aside for the intensive caring and treatment of dying patients with special problems, usually including severe pain. It is like a minihospice within a general hospital setting. The PCU allows patients to return home and stay home with family and friends in more familiar surroundings for as long as possible. The PCU has formed a Palliative Care Service that goes beyond the hospital itself: it extends its services to the home.

The pain clinic and the hospice are breakthroughs of the highest importance in the clinical management of pain. We can be thankful that pain doctors and researchers have been blessed by God with the ability to achieve such breakthroughs, and we can hope for more to come in the years ahead.

Part Two

Spiritual Responses to Pain

7

Pain & Healing:
The Power of God

TIM IS A FORTY-FIVE-YEAR-OLD WHO IS BRANCH MANAGER OF A major bank in his city. His job requires him to attend many meetings and often involves working overtime, including some weekends. He enjoys his work despite the stressful and demanding schedule he has to keep. However, in the past few years it has become increasingly difficult for him to work such long hours, primarily because he has been suffering from arthritis. He often has pain, sometimes intense and even excruciating pain, in his joints, particularly in his elbow and wrist areas. He has been taking pain medications as well as medication for arthritis, but his pain has persisted.

Tim is a Christian. He has been an elder in his church for over ten years. He is actively involved in leading a men's small group that meets weekly and teaching adult Sunday school on Sundays. In the past year, Tim has been studying the Bible in more depth regarding what it actually teaches about the healing power of God. He has also attended a couple of renewal meetings conducted by speakers who are involved in healing ministries. He has been blessed at such meetings, as he has requested prayer for the healing of his arthritis and the associated joint pain, as well as for more of the filling and power of the Holy Spirit in his life and ministry as a Christian. Prayer-team members at these meetings prayed intensely for him, and he testifies that as a result he is experiencing deeper intimacy with God, spending more time in prayer and reading the Bible daily. He also has a greater burden for the lost, praying for them and seeking out opportunities, intentionally and prayerfully, to share the gospel with them. He believes that God has touched him more deeply in his spiritual life.

Tim's arthritis pain has recently begun to subside in intensity as well as frequency. He therefore is thankful to God for allowing him to experience more of his healing power. Tim is trusting and praying that God will heal his arthritis and pain even more fully in the near future. He has continued to ask for prayer ministry from friends and his pastors, as well as from prayer-ministry team members at special healing or renewal meetings that he still attends when they are organized in his city.

Tim's recent experience of partial healing of his arthritis pain and inflammation in his elbow and wrist joint areas, and his hope for more complete healing soon, raise a number of important questions regarding what the Bible has to say about pain and the healing power of God. For example, are supernatural healings or healing miracles possible today? If so, how often do they take place? How do we pray for and receive such healing? Does healing *always* occur if we have enough faith in the power of God? Or is it more a matter of God's sovereign choice, so that he decides who gets healed and who doesn't?

These important questions about pain and healing focusing on the power of God working in our lives today need to be discussed further in this chapter, before I go on to describe several spiritual methods or means of pain control from a Christian perspective in the next chapter. Like Tim and many other Christians, you may be wondering what you can realistically expect from God if you pray for him to heal you of your chronic-pain condition or other physical illnesses.

Is Healing Possible Today?

Many Christian books have been written in recent years on the topic of the healing power of God.[1] Many of them will answer this question affirmatively and conclude that supernatural healings or healing miracles are definitely possible today.

The Bible portrays God as Healer throughout both the Old and New Testaments. As John Wimber, pastor and founder of the Vineyard churches, has pointed out, the Gospels contain twenty-six accounts of individuals being healed physically, and the book of Acts contains five. Jesus Christ in his earthly ministry often healed the sick and cast out demons (see, for example, Mk 1:34). He also commissioned the twelve apostles (Lk 9:1) and the seventy-two disciples (Lk 10:9) to do likewise—to conduct a healing ministry. However, physical healing is mentioned only sporadically in the Epistles in the New Testament (for example, see 1 Cor 12:8-11, 28-30). And James 5:13-16 is the only direct passage in the New Testament that tells us how to go about praying for the sick.[2] Depending on how one interprets these passages in the Bible, two somewhat different versions of the affirmative answer to the question of whether healing miracles occur today are possible.

The first version, represented by authors like John Wimber and Dr. Peter Wagner, professor of church growth in the School of World Mission at Fuller Theological Seminary, is an enthusiastic endorsement of healing ministries today. This view would see supernatural healings as a significant part of the ministry that Jesus has called all Christians to do in his name and that some specially gifted Christians have the spiritual gifts to particularly focus on. The answer, therefore, to whether healing miracles take place today is a definite and strong "Yes!"

The second version, represented by authors like Dr. Colin Brown, professor of systematic theology and associate dean, Center for Advanced Theological Studies at Fuller Theological Seminary, is a more guarded and cautious affirmation of healing miracles today. This view would see supernatural healings as periodic occurrences that can and do take place, but not as frequently as some may claim. They are also viewed as *not* as central to the mission and ministry to which Jesus has called Christians. His mission for his followers today has to do more with preaching the gospel—the good news of salvation, forgiveness of sins, peace with God and the assurance of eternal life through his death and resurrection—than with supernatural physical healing per se.

Also, Dr. Brown would urge us to refrain from calling all kinds of physical improvements in answer to prayer "miracles." He would suggest reserving the term for supernatural acts of the Holy Spirit in bringing about instant and complete cures of physical illnesses. Other partial healings or smaller-scale improvements in physical health should be more appropriately called "answers to prayer." Brown does agree that God is still active today in healing ministries and that supernatural healings or healing miracles can and do occur, but rather infrequently. More often, we receive many smaller answers to prayer for physical healing.

I believe that based on a careful study of the Bible and the writings of authors like these, it is safe and biblical to conclude that God still heals today; healing miracles can and do take place. The next question has to do with how often they occur, and there are some different opinions here. Some will say they occur quite often and would take place even more frequently if we learned to exercise more faith in praying more for healing miracles in the name of Jesus and according to God's will. Others will say they occur somewhat infrequently, and what happens more often are smaller-scale healings that are not really miraculous, but they are still God's gracious answers to prayer for healing. Perhaps it is not critical how we answer this question of frequency. The more crucial question for people suffering from chronic-pain conditions or other physical illness is, *How do we pray for and receive physical healings from God, whether they be complete and instant healing miracles or smaller-scale healings?*

Ministering the Whole Gospel

While Jesus has called those of us who are Christians and therefore his disciples to primarily carry out his Great Commission of sharing the gospel with unbelievers and making them disciples as well (Mt 28:18-20), he has also called us who believe in him to minister to people and do his works, and even greater works (Jn 14:12), as his Holy Spirit empowers us (Acts 1:8). "His works" definitely include healing and setting people free from demonic bondage. We can therefore pray for physical as well as emotional or inner healing as part of the ministry he has called us to do.

The Lord's heart of compassion for lost, broken and hurting people will motivate us to minister to them in every way, including praying for physical healing (without losing sight of the primacy of their finding salvation through accepting Jesus Christ personally as Lord and Savior). We also must not forget the importance of social justice and social action—motivated by the same compassion of Jesus and the power of the Holy Spirit—in overcoming societal evils like racism, injustice, sexism, political and economic oppression. With this bigger picture in mind, we can now move on to consider how to go about praying for and receiving physical healing for chronic-pain conditions in particular.

Praying for Your Own Physical Healing

First of all, you can begin by praying for yourself and your pain problem. However, it is crucial that we come to the Lord with the *right heart motive:* to seek him and his will for us first, rather than simply to demand healing from him so that we can feel good and be relieved of pain. We need to ask ourselves *why* we are asking or praying for physical healing. It should be for God's glory and to serve him and others better as he gives us health and strength. And we need to submit to his will, so that if he chooses *not* to heal us, we will accept his answer with grace and trust that he knows best and in all things works for our good ultimately (Rom 8:28). I will deal with this issue of suffering and grace in more detail in a later chapter.

Mark 1:32-34 describes how crowds of people in a city began coming to Jesus for healing of those sick with various illnesses and diseases and for casting out of demons from those who were demonized or demon-possessed. In commenting on this text, Dr. William Barclay writes the following, emphasizing again the need to have a *right heart motive* for coming to Jesus for healing—with a heart of love for him:

> But there is the beginning of tragedy here. The crowds came . . . because *they wanted something out of Jesus.* They did not come because they loved Him. . . . In the last analysis they wanted to use Him. . . . We must all go to Jesus for He alone can give us the things we need for life; but if that going, and these gifts do not produce in us an answering love and gratitude, there is something tragically wrong. God is not someone to be used in the day of misfortune; He is someone to be loved and remembered every day of our lives.[3]

We need, therefore, to come to Jesus with hearts that will love *him* more than his blessings. We need to learn to love the Giver more than the gifts, the Healer more than the healing, the Deliverer more than the deliverance! However, there are times when a Christian who suffers excruciating pain may be angry at God for "allowing" the pain to be so bad and to persist. He or she may therefore cry out to God for help and healing with an attitude that is not right or humble. God is so merciful and full of grace that he still often answers such cries or prayers, granting some relief, if not complete healing, to those who suffer terrible pain that persists but who also struggle with negative attitudes toward him.

Nevertheless, it is better to come to the Lord with a right heart motive or attitude of love for him alone and concern only for his will to be done and his glory to be manifested. You can then proceed to pray for healing of your chronic pain. The following is a sample prayer you can use.

> Dear Lord, you know that I have been suffering from this chronic pain condition [specify what it is, e.g., headaches, low-back pain]

for quite some time now. I have tried medical treatments and other methods of pain control, with little help. I humble myself before you and seek you first. I'm deeply thankful to you for saving me eternally and forgiving me of my sins because of your finished work on the cross, where you died for me and the world, and your resurrection as Victor over death, sin and Satan.

I come to you right now asking that you will release your healing power, by the Holy Spirit. Please touch my body where it hurts so badly and so often, and heal my pain condition. Release me from the pain so that I can love you and serve you better. I receive your healing power and wholeness now by faith, and I trust you to continue healing me of my pain. I submit myself to you and your will for me. Thank you for listening and ministering to me with your love and grace and healing power. I claim your victory over the works of the devil. I love you, Lord, and worship you! I pray all these things in the powerful name of Jesus Christ, my Lord and Savior. Amen!

You can also add a prayer for the Lord to bless any medical or other treatments for pain control that you may be using. For example, you may pray,

Dear Lord, I also ask in the name of Jesus that you release your healing power through the medical and other treatments I am using for pain control. You are ultimately the source of all true healing, and you work in and through many different ways, including medicine and other pain treatments. Please bless these treatments and grant me more pain relief through them, and through your healing touch, for your honor and glory. In Jesus' name I pray, with thanksgiving. Amen!

Whatever happens, remember *never* to stop taking medication without first consulting your physician or pain specialist. Pain medications usually need to be tapered off gradually, if you have been on them for a long time.

Second, you can also ask for prayer from your pastor, church leaders or close friends, especially those who may have the *spiritual gift of healing*. Dr. Wagner defines this gift as follows.

> The gift of healing is the special ability that God gives to certain members of the Body of Christ to serve as human intermediaries through whom it pleases God to cure illnesses and restore health apart from the use of natural means.[4]

Praying for Another Person's Healing

Christians with the spiritual gift of healing are enabled by the power of the Holy Spirit to pray for healing usually or often with positive results. However, medical and other relevant help or treatments for physical illnesses and pain conditions should still be used. Prayer for healing through such "natural" means is also needed.

Such prayer times can of course occur privately; they can also occur informally, between you and your pastor, church leaders or friends. Or they can be more formal, involving the church leaders. James 5:14-16 provides the following instructions for special prayer for the sick:

> Is any one of you sick? He should call the elders of the church to pray over him and anoint him with oil in the name of the Lord. And the prayer offered in faith will make the sick person well; the Lord will raise him up. If he has sinned, he will be forgiven. There- fore confess your sins to each other and pray for each other so that you may be healed. The prayer of a righteous man is powerful and effective.

The sick person (including the person with a chronic-pain condition) can either call the elders (or pastors or church leaders) to the home for such prayer offered in faith for healing, with the anointing with oil in the Lord's name, or go to a special healing service at the church, if there is one, where the elders and pastors will gather together to pray for the sick, following the instructions in James 5:14-16. James emphasizes the need to confess our sins to each other as we pray for the healing of one another's sicknesses. Some churches have special prayer-ministry teams available after a church service to pray for people with different needs, including those who need physical healing of various illnesses and pain conditions. It should be noted that some Bible scholars are of the opinion that the anointing with oil in the original context and culture was more medicinal than sacramental. Oil was used as a medicine and healing agent in those days. It reminds us that *both prayer and medicine* (or other natural healing methods) are important in physical healing.

When Healing Does Not Come

Can we expect that physical healing will always occur if we have enough faith in God's power? What about the sovereignty of God?

James 5:14-16 emphasizes the importance of the prayer of *faith* in bringing about physical healing of the sick. Other passages in the New Testament also indicate the need for faith as the means through which God releases his healing power (see Mt 8:5-13; Lk 8:48; 17:19; 18:42; Acts 3:16; 14:9-10).

John Wimber has pointed out that such faith is exercised not only by the sick person needing physical healing (as in Mk 5:34) but also by friends or relatives of the sick (as in Mk 2:5; 5:36) as well as by those who pray for the healing of the sick (Mk 9:14-29). Therefore, while faith is needed, it is *not* essential that such faith be the faith the sick person has in the healing power of God. *It is cruel and wrong, when a sick person is not healed after prayer for physical healing is offered, to blame that person for his or her lack of faith.* Such blaming is often done in some Christian circles. Whose faith then is most important for divine healing—the faith of the sick person, friends, relatives or those who pray for healing? Wimber suggests that "*anyone* who has faith" in Jesus for miracles can be used by God to release his healing power.[5]

Does this mean that if there is *enough faith,* whatever the source, then physical healing will *always* take place? What about the sovereignty of God and his mysterious will that we don't always understand, such that it is ultimately God who chooses who gets healed and who doesn't?

It is actually clear from Scripture that not everyone is healed, even if faith is abundant and prayers are offered in faith many times for physical healing. For example, Epaphroditus (Phil 2:27), Timothy (1 Tim 5:23), Trophimus (2 Tim 4:20) and the apostle Paul himself (2 Cor 12:7-10; Gal 4:13-14) were not healed immediately, and in some of these cases, such as Timothy and Paul, they possibly were never healed. Having enough faith, therefore, does *not* guarantee physical healing. The sovereignty of God ultimately rules over all our experiences on earth, including experiences of physical healing. We need to come humbly to God and ask for his healing—but then yield to his will alone.

Again, we need to desire God more than just physical healing. Sometimes he doesn't heal, as in the case of Paul's thorn in the flesh, which some Bible scholars, like Colin Brown, say probably referred to Paul's defective eyesight (Gal 4:13-14). In such cases God has promised grace sufficient to bear the physical condition or pain (2 Cor 12:7-10). In other words, we need to have a clear biblical perspective on both healing and the power of God, as well as on suffering and the grace of God.

Wimber suggests, however, that *most* (not all) of the reasons people are not healed even after being prayed for involve some form of sin and unbelief. Such reasons include not having faith in God for healing (Jas 5:15); personal, unconfessed sin that is a barrier to God's grace (Jas 5:16); continuing disunity, sin and unbelief within Christian groups, churches or families that hinder healing in individual members of the body of Christ (1 Cor 11:30); incomplete or inaccurate diagnoses so that people do not know how to pray correctly; and assuming that God always heals immediately, so that when instant healing doesn't occur, people stop praying prematurely.[6]

He also points out that most physical healing is a process that takes time. This is because other factors—emotional, psychological or demonic—may need to be dealt with first, before the physical healing can occur.[7] There are times, therefore, when other help may also be necessary: counseling, inner-healing prayer or prayer for healing of

traumatic memories, or prayer for deliverance from demonic afflic-
tion (demonization) or exorcism, and not simply prayer for physical
healing.

The physical healing of chronic-pain conditions can therefore still
take place today, as a demonstration or manifestation of God's healing power. While further study is still needed, a recent review on
prayer and health concluded that empirical research partially con-
firms that prayer promotes a variety of health outcomes.[8] However,
ultimately, as we pray in faith for healing and health, we also need
to submit to God's sovereign will and seek him first—above and
beyond the healing itself.

8

Spiritual Means of Pain Control

T HE PREVIOUS CHAPTER DISCUSSED THE HEALING POWER OF GOD that can help to significantly reduce or even remove chronic-pain conditions and other illnesses. There are several specific spiritual means of pain control that Christians can use to manage chronic pain more effectively.

Prayer
As already described in the previous chapter, prayer can be a very helpful and powerful spiritual means of pain control. Specific prayer for physical healing of chronic-pain conditions can be offered by the person suffering from pain, by his or her close friends or family members, or by church leaders (pastors, elders) or prayer ministry teams.

Recently I attended and spoke at a "Service for Healing and Wholeness" at La Canada Presbyterian Church in the Los Angeles area, where my good friend Rev. Dr. Chuck Osburn serves as associate pastor for pastoral care and counseling and directs a very significant lay counseling ministry. I also participated in praying for the sick, including some who were suffering from pain. It was a great service, deeply blessed by the Lord, and I was blessed myself as I took part in it. Prayer for healing of the sick through special worship and healing services can and should be conducted more often. The following is one example of how it can be done, as practiced at La Canada Presbyterian Church and described in their monthly church bulletin for the Service for Healing and Wholeness.

The LCPC [La Canada Presbyterian Church] Congregational Care Committee continually asks the question "How can we better care for the people of our congregation and community?" As one part of the answer to that question, we recognize a growing need and desire by members of our church and community to have more opportunities for special prayer for those who are sick and hurting.

The Biblical admonition is clear: "Is any one of you in trouble? You should pray. . . . Is any one of you sick [hurting, depressed, physically ill, relationally broken, feeling alienated from God, etc.]? You should call the elders of the church to pray over you and anoint you with oil" (Jas 5).

In response, the Session of our Church unanimously approved the Congregational Care Committee's proposal to begin monthly worship services that allow time and focus for the personal needs of individuals to be brought forward for prayer by our Pastors and Elders.

The order of worship for this service has been taken from our Presbyterian Church (USA)'s Supplemental Manual for Pastoral Care. We will sing a variety of hymns and songs, hear a Meditation, offer the Lord's Supper, and following the Biblical direction of James 5, we will invite people to be prayed for, offering the practice of the laying on of hands and anointing with oil.

This service is open to all and we encourage everyone to come to be prayed for, as well as to participate in the privilege and loving act of prayer for others.

If you have a chronic-pain condition and happen to attend a church that has a similar worship and healing service, you may find it helpful

and a real blessing to attend such a service and receive prayer for
healing by the pastors, elders or other prayer ministry leaders. If your
church does not have a formal service where prayer for healing of
the sick is a major focus, you can still ask your church's pastors, elders
or leaders to pray for you. This can be done, usually with the anointing with oil (more sacramentally than medicinally today), either in the
privacy of your home or at a special prayer time for you at the church.

I have been describing prayer so far in terms of specific requests
for physical healing, including healing of chronic-pain conditions.
However, prayer is bigger than simply asking for healing. Prayer has
many dimensions: it includes at least confession, adoration or praise,
thanksgiving, petition (or requests for oneself) and intercession (or
praying for others). Prayer is simply communion with God and includes being quiet or silent in solitude and simply waiting on him,
worshiping him and listening to him. I have heard testimonies from
pain patients who have experienced complete or at least temporary
or partial relief of their pain while worshiping God—in prayer or
singing, individually or corporately—during a service. They have also
often experienced deep joy and peace. Prayer has helped many to cast
their cares on the Lord and *suffer less* from their pain, even if their
actual pain experience did not change much. In particular, prayer
with thanksgiving can help you overcome anxiety and experience the
peace of God that transcends all understanding (Phil 4:6-7), thereby
enabling you to have more effective pain control.

Dr. Richard Foster has written an excellent book on prayer; it describes twenty-one different types of prayer! He also offers the following loving invitation from God to all of us—to spend more time in
prayer, so that intimacy with God can help put many things in our
lives, including pain experiences, in proper perspective.

God has graciously allowed me to catch a glimpse into his heart,
and I want to share with you what I have seen. Today the heart
of God is an open wound of love. He aches over our distance and
preoccupation. He mourns that we do not draw near to Him. He

grieves that we have forgotten Him. He weeps over our obsession with muchness and manyness. He longs for our presence.

And He is inviting you—and me—to come home, to come home where we belong, to come home to that for which we were created. His arms are stretched out wide to receive us. His heart is enlarged to take us in.

For too long we have been in a far country: a country of noise and hurry and crowds, a country of climb and push and shove, a country of frustration and fear and intimidation. And He welcomes us home: Home to serenity and peace and joy, home to friendship and fellowship and openness, home to intimacy and acceptance and affirmation.

. . . The key to this home, this heart of God, is prayer.[1]

Solitude and Private Retreats

In addition to regular times of prayer daily, longer periods of solitude alone with God or in private retreats can also be particularly helpful to you if you are a Christian suffering from chronic pain. Foster has some very good insights and suggestions regarding such private retreats or special times of solitude.

Have you ever noticed the many times Jesus experienced solitude? Mark's haunting words, "in the morning, a great while before day, he arose and went out to a lonely place," is the signature written across Jesus' ministry (1:35). Jesus needed frequent retreat and solitude to do his work, and yet somehow we think we can get by without the same. It is time we follow our Leader's lead.

The major thing a private retreat accomplishes is to create an open empty space in our lives. We learn to "waste" time for God. Slowly, we come to hear God's speech in his wondrous, terrible, loving, all-embracing silence. Gently we press into the holy of holies where we are sifted in the stillness. Painfully, we let go of the vain images of ourselves that seemed so essential. Joyfully, we loosen our grip on all those projects that appeared so significant.

Most wonderful of all is the empowerment we receive: Overcoming love, faith that can see everything in the light of God's governance for good, hope that can carry us through the most discouraging of circumstances, and power to overcome evil and do what is right.

I urge every one . . . to experience a private retreat at least once a year. A weekend is a wonderful time frame . . . you will need to schedule such times far ahead, otherwise competing commitments will eat you alive.

. . . First, choose a place that is free from distraction. Go to a retreat center that understands what a private retreat is and will honor your need for silence. Or perhaps you can find a mountain cabin, or a beach house.

Second, stoutly refuse to over-structure the time. Long prayer-filled walks are often more useful than hectic-filled rituals. Quiet meditation on a single phrase of Scripture is frequently preferable to panting through many chapters. Reflecting in a journal on the work of God within us is usually more profitable than massive reading of devotional literature. Sometimes nothing should be done—simply and intentionally "waste" time for God. Happy retreating![2]

Such occasional times of prolonged solitude, even if only for half a day or a day (and in your own home if it is not practical for you to take a day or two off to go to a special retreat center or other quiet place), can be blessed times of communion with God. As Foster has pointed out, "wasting" time for God can help you to experience God's power and love in such a way that you will be enabled to see things with the eyes of faith from God's perspective and deepen in hope, knowing more certainly that he will work things out eventually for your own good (Rom 8:28). He will help you to cope more effectively with the trials and difficulties of your life, including your struggle with chronic pain, by increasing your faith and hope in him.

In fact, Paul Brand and Philip Yancey have noted that in a survey (conducted by the late Norman Cousins) of 649 oncologists or cancer specialists, more than 90 percent of them attached the highest value to attitudes of *hope* and *optimism* in their patients.[3] Solitude and private retreats can help you to deepen your communion with God, and that will help you grow in faith and hope, even when at times God doesn't seem to make sense in the context of the difficult circumstances and trials of your life, including pain. Dr. James Dobson has written *When God Doesn't Make Sense,* which you may find to be of real help and blessing.[4]

Other Spiritual Disciplines

Foster has actually described a total of twelve spiritual disciplines that can help Christians grow spiritually and know God more deeply, becoming more like Jesus in the process. In his classic book *Celebration of Discipline* he describes the following spiritual disciplines: the *inward disciplines* of meditation, prayer, fasting and study; the *outward disciplines* of solitude, submission, simplicity and service; and the *corporate disciplines* of confession, worship, guidance and celebration.[5]

The regular practice of these spiritual disciplines, empowered by the Holy Spirit, can help you to experience God more intimately—and to cope more effectively with your chronic-pain condition.

Meditation on Scripture

I would like to describe in more detail the spiritual discipline of meditation on Scripture. It is a crucial means to knowing God's Word more deeply and thereby to gaining a more meaningful and eternal perspective on life and its varied experiences.

Foster describes meditation on Scripture as centering on internalizing and personalizing particular verses or passages in such a way that the written Word of God, the Bible, becomes a living word given for you. The use of the imagination to let the Word of God come alive may be particularly helpful. Meditation is therefore different from study of Scripture, which focuses more on exegesis and interpretation of the text or passage under consideration. Foster also suggests that in meditation we should *not* try to pass over many Bible passages quickly and superficially. Instead, we need to choose one verse or simple text and try to live with it throughout the day.

David Ray some years ago wrote a helpful book on the art of Christian meditation, in which he suggested the following steps.

1. Select your *word for the day* (e.g., *peace*) and use a meditation card that provides a *definition* of the word (e.g., peace: a state of tranquility; freedom from mental agitation, fear and anger; harmony) and a *Bible verse* to meditate on (e.g., Jn 14:27: "Peace I [Jesus] leave with you; my peace I give you. . . . Do not let your hearts be troubled, and do not be afraid").

2. Get in a *comfortable and relaxed position*.

3. Repeat your *meditation cue* two or three times by bringing to mind verses such as Psalm 46:10, Isaiah 26:3 or Isaiah 40:31.

4. Use *conscious thought* to slowly and deliberately look at your meditation card; think carefully and intently about your word, its definition and particularly the Bible verse.

5. *Close your eyes* gently and softly to communicate with God more personally.

6. Use *mental pictures* or imagery to let the Bible verse come alive (e.g., imagining Jesus standing beside you, speaking to you directly and bestowing his peace upon you, and yourself receiving him and his peace with thanksgiving).

7. *Pray*, conversing with God openly, sharing with him your every thought and feeling.

8. *Open your eyes* as you end your time of meditation on Scripture, which should typically take about fifteen minutes a day according to Ray.[6]

Dr. Jay Adams has pointed out that biblical meditation on Scripture is different from Transcendental Meditation (TM) and other Eastern mystical forms of meditation. Christian or biblical meditation focuses intensively, with the heart, on *biblical truth* and not on the self.

Adams notes that the two main words for *meditation* in the Bible actually mean "to murmur or mutter" and "to speak to one's self." Meditation, therefore, is a process of focused, concentrated inner thinking or reasoning that Adams points out will eventually result in outward action that is pleasing to God. He teaches that part of one's meditation is thinking carefully through a verse or text from Scripture, with the following questions suggested by Adams: "What does it mean to me? How will it change my life? What are some concrete things that I must do about it? How can I get these things accomplished?"[7]

Adams, therefore, emphasizes the *active* side of biblical meditation, whereas other authors have emphasized the need to be quiet and passive or *detached* from the hustle and bustle of the world and daily living, so as to be *attached* to God and his Word more deeply. Christian meditation, however, is vastly different from other forms of meditation that focus only on the emptying of one's mind or detachment from the world.

Meditation on Scripture, as well as Scripture memory (memorizing specific Bible verses, especially those that may have special meaning for you), can be of great help to you as you take time to let God's Word—God's eternal truth—touch you deeply, enabling you to trust him and rest in him more and thereby putting your chronic pain and other life experiences in proper perspective. You may therefore find meaning in your suffering from pain, such that your suffering may be eased.

The spiritual implications of the experience of chronic pain, however, can differ from patient to patient. William Conwill describes three major traditional views of pain that you can take: (1) *pain as punishment* from God for some wrong attitude or act; (2) *pain as an opportunity for transcendence* by accepting God's wisdom and humbly submitting to the suffering and pain as part of purification of the godly, thus transcending the pain; (3) *pain as redemptive salvific activity*, or helping and saving others through one's own pain. He also notes that a pain patient's religious interpretation of his or her pain can be *conventional* (characteristic of the denomination or religious group of which the patient is a member), *idiosyncratic* (reasonable and realistic but more personal to the patient) or *bizarre* (not clearly connected with reality and somewhat delusional or even hallucinatory in nature).[8]

Dr. Avie Rainwater has pointed out that while many pain patients experience living with pain as spiritually awakening, they also often express struggles with doubts and feeling betrayed by God, and they seldom see pain as something positive sent by God.[9] Whatever your spiritual beliefs or interpretations concerning your chronic-pain experience, it is important to have a personal theology, based on meditating on Scripture, that focuses on God's grace and love for you. Your hope and trust in God's faithfulness, his goodness, his forgiveness and his ultimately working all things out for your own good (including healing if that is his will for you) can help you to actually suffer less from your pain, perhaps by closing more of the pain gates in your central nervous system through descending neural influences or nerve pathways.[10]

Fellowship and Worship

You may also find regular times of *fellowship*, meeting with other fellow Christians in small groups or relatively larger church groups, to be helpful for achieving better pain control. Through such times of mutual support, sharing, prayer and often Bible study, you can experience comfort and encouragement from others. And you can focus your attention on them and the activities of the fellowship or small group you are attending, thus distracting yourself from your pain. A special kind of support group or small group can also be organized for chronic-pain sufferers, who agree to meet regularly (weekly, biweekly or even monthly) to share their pain experiences in an understanding and empathic way, to compare coping methods and to pray for each other. The benefits and blessings of a caring and loving community or fellowship are potentially great and can help you to manage chronic pain more effectively.

Some people with chronic pain have also found their regular times of *worship* particularly helpful. These times may be their own quiet times alone with God or corporate experiences—a church Sunday worship service, the worship segment of a fellowship or small group, or a devotional time with a spouse or family. Such worship times usually include the singing of hymns or praise songs, or listening to worship music, and prayers of thanksgiving and praise to God—all of which can help lift up your spirit and enable you to experience deeper intimacy with God. A common result is that you may also have less intense pain during these times of worship.

Trusting God and having a biblical, Christian perspective on life, suffering and eternity can be particularly helpful in living effectively with chronic pain. There are times, however, when the pain persists even after you have tried all possible methods or means of pain control. It is especially important at such times to focus more on the grace of God that enables us to live with persistent pain and suffering. The next chapter will cover this crucial topic.

9

Pain & Suffering: The Grace of God

O NE OF THE MOST DIFFICULT QUESTIONS FOR A PERSON SUFFER-
ing from a chronic-pain condition that persists in its intensity
and duration is "Why doesn't the pain go away?" This is especially
true if all kinds of pain management methods have been tried, including spiritual means of pain control. For a Christian suffering from such
persistent pain, the question may become what Philip Yancey has entitled his excellent and helpful book *Where Is God When It Hurts?*[1]

The problem of personal suffering and the bigger problem of evil
in this fallen, sinful world in which we live are twin questions that do
not have simple answers. It is a fact that not all chronic-pain conditions or other sicknesses get healed in answer to prayers for healing
and relief. As I pointed out in chapter seven, God does not always
heal, even if we ask for healing in prayer with great faith. We do not
always understand his will or his ways of working; at times God does
not make sense to us.

Where Is God in All This?
When pain continues at almost unbearable and excruciating levels of
intensity, we may even feel deep emotional hurt and disappointment

with God. Philip Yancey has also written an insightful book on just such a theme of disappointment with God, focusing on three key questions: Is God unfair? Is God silent? Is God hidden?[2] Often we may feel he is unfair, silent and hidden in the struggle against chronic pain that persists as badly as ever.

Yancey's basic answer to why a loving God can allow such terrible suffering to happen is centered in God's desire to have a passionate, loving relationship with his people. God wants to be loved—not analyzed! He also wants us to experience his great love for us, even in the midst of pain that does not seem to let up. This requires what Yancey calls *fidelity*, which is a deeper, more mysterious kind of faith that has learned to trust God no matter how things may appear. This kind of faith, the *deepest faith* or *fidelity*, according to Yancey, seems to develop best when things are unclear or foggy, when God remains silent in the midst of deep pain and great loss or overwhelming, traumatic disappointment, as in the case of Job.

Job lost seven thousand sheep, three thousand camels, five thousand oxen, five hundred donkeys, as well as many servants and all of his seven sons and three daughters. He also lost his health, breaking out with painful sores from head to toe. Glandion Carney and William Long recently wrote a book also based on Job, entitled *Trusting God Again*, on regaining hope after disappointment and loss. They aptly describe Job's struggle thus: "When he then experienced the tremendous dislocation and loss of family, wealth and health, Job was not simply disoriented by the loss and wracked by pain. He felt that his most basic understanding of God and God's character was at stake. Certainly he could expect pain in this life, but *this much pain?* Certainly loss is a real part of human experience, but *such overwhelming loss?*"[3]

You may have feelings and questions like Job's as you struggle with chronic pain that doesn't go away.

Our Wounded Surgeon
Ultimately, Yancey's answer to the question "Where is God when it

hurts?" points us to the cross and to Jesus Christ, who suffered and died for us and rose again that we may have hope and salvation. He writes: "The surgery of life hurts. It helps me, though, to know that the surgeon himself, the Wounded Surgeon, has felt every stab of pain and every sorrow."[4]

If you are suffering from a pain condition that seems to be getting no better and may even be getting worse, you may find the following concluding statements from Yancey helpful and hope-filled.

Where is God when it hurts?

He has been there from the beginning, designing a pain system that, even in the midst of a fallen world, still bears the stamp of his genius and equips us for life on this planet.

He transforms pain, using it to teach and strengthen us, if we allow it to turn us toward him.

With great restraint, he watches this rebellious planet live on, in mercy allowing the human project to continue in its self-guided way.

He lets us cry out like Job, in loud fits of anger against him, blaming him for a world we spoiled.

He allies himself with the poor and suffering, founding a kingdom tilted in their favor. He stoops to conquer.

He has joined us. He has hurt and bled and cried and suffered. He has dignified for all time those who suffer, by sharing their pain.

He is with us now, ministering to us through his Spirit and through members of his body who are commissioned to bear us up and relieve our suffering for the sake of the head.

He is waiting, gathering the armies of good. One day he will unleash them, and the world will see one last terrifying moment of suffering before the full victory is ushered in. Then, God will create for us a new, incredible world. And pain shall be no more.[5]

Yancey drew these conclusions based on the Bible, God's Word. They can help you cope better with chronic pain that doesn't improve by giving you hope and pointing you to the grace of God that will always be sufficient for your every need. The apostle Paul did not experience relief from his "thorn in the flesh," his physical impediment, but God gave him grace sufficient for him to bear it and made his own power perfect in Paul's weakness. Paul therefore concluded: "For when I am weak, then I am strong" (2 Cor 12:9-10).

God does not always promise miraculous healing for our pain and suffering. But he always promises grace sufficient for our every need, enabling us to endure the pain and suffering. As a result, we grow to become better people, more like Christ in every way, through the pain and suffering that cause us to be more humble and dependent on God.

As Dr. Ellie Sturgis has stated: "The New Testament view of suffering as depicted in 1 Peter is that suffering is a means of purifying or ennobling the soul, bringing us into closer fellowship with Christ and leading to a more harmonious life in congruence with God's will."[6]

Sturgis also points out that it is more helpful and biblical not to view God as only punitive and pain as a punishment, thereby reducing one's motivation for change and frustrating rehabilitation efforts. Rather, God should be more accurately seen as forgiving and an ever present source of support and strength,[7] although sometimes in this life he may seem to be silent, hidden and even unfair.

The Uses of Pain

It is true that at times God can use pain as his way of disciplining or chastening us (Heb 12:5-6) so that we will pay more attention to him and turn from our sinful ways to deeper obedience and love for him. For example, David experienced searing pain in his back and wounds that festered and were loathsome, as well as feeling feeble and utterly crushed, with anguish of heart, because of his self-acknowledged sinful folly (see Ps 38, especially verses 5-8, 17-18). However, it is still God's love for us that is behind such discipline, and not harshness or punitive punishment per se. God does not enjoy seeing us suffer.

He brings good out of evil, out of our suffering (Gen 50:20), because of his goodness and grace.

At other times, pain has nothing to do with being disciplined or chastened for our own good. It may simply be part of his pruning work as a loving Gardener in our lives, to produce even more spiritual fruit in a life that is already abiding in Christ and bearing fruit! (Jn 15:1-8).

And there are times when our suffering and pain are used by God to bring blessing and salvation to others (see 2 Cor 1:3-7). Therefore, there is always meaning in our suffering and pain, even though we may not see it yet. Most of all, the Lord is with us—he has suffered for us (Heb 5:8) and he suffers again with us (Heb 4:15), being able to sympathize with our weaknesses and struggles. You can therefore go to him boldly in prayer, approaching his throne of grace with confidence that you will receive mercy and find grace to help you in your time of need (Heb 4:16).

Pain Caused by the Enemy
It should be pointed out, however, that at times physical suffering and pain may actually be the direct work or attack of Satan against us as God's people. Satan, the devil, is our adversary, our enemy who seeks to devour and destroy us if possible (1 Pet 5:8). There is spiritual warfare present in our lives (Eph 6:10-18). Therefore, we are to put on the armor of God and use prayer and the Word of God especially to stand against the devil's attacks, resisting him so he will flee from us (Jas 4:7). In the book of Job we read clearly that Satan was the one responsible for smiting Job with painful sores from the soles of his feet to the top of his head (2:7) as well as wiping out his wealth, his possessions, and his sons and daughters (1:16, 19). Yet Satan could not do any of this evil without first being permitted by God (1:12; 2:6). God is still sovereign and ultimately in control, although he does not cause evil per se.

Not only does God's grace enable and strengthen us sufficiently to endure pain and suffering in this life and to overcome satanic attacks, but his grace also gives us an absolute hope and certain promise of the life to come! Through the death and resurrection of Jesus Christ and our faith in receiving him personally into our hearts as our Lord and Savior, we have assurance of eternal life and heaven to come forever (Jn 1:12; 1 Jn 5:11-12). The apostle Paul therefore states in Romans 8:18: "I consider that our present sufferings are not worth comparing with the glory that will be revealed in us." And in 2 Corinthians 4:17-18: "For our light and momentary troubles are achieving for us an eternal glory that far outweighs them all. So we fix our eyes not on what is seen, but on what is unseen. For what is seen is temporary, but what is unseen is eternal."

It has often been said, "Don't be so heavenly minded that you are of no earthly good!" However, it will help you to cope better with chronic pain that persists if you learn to be heavenly minded enough—by faith and fidelity, like Paul—to continue to be of earthly good!

The ultimate promise of heaven to come that is particularly encouraging and relevant for chronic pain sufferers is found in Revelation 21:4: "He will wipe every tear from their eyes. There will be no more death or mourning or crying or pain, for the old order of things has passed away." That day shall come soon when all pain and suffering will be gone forever, thank God! The Lord Jesus is coming back again soon to bring ultimate relief and eternal life fully to those of us who are believers and his disciples. Death (and pain) shall be finally conquered (1 Cor 15:51-55)! As Yancey puts it: "In any discussion of disappointment with God, heaven is the last word, the most important word of all. Only heaven will finally solve the problem of God's hiddenness. For the first time ever, human beings will be able to look upon God face to face. In the midst of his agony, Job somehow came up with faith to believe that 'in my flesh I will see God; I myself will see him with my own eyes.' That prophecy will come true not just for Job but for all of us."[8]

Daily Grace

God's grace is available day by day to help you live with pain and suffering and manage your chronic pain in the best ways possible. Pain and suffering, however, will remain somewhat of a mystery, one that we will not solve or understand fully until we are in heaven. There may therefore be times when your pain is so bad that all you can do is to cry out to God as Job did.

> Terrors overwhelm me;
>> my dignity is driven away as by the wind,
>> my safety vanishes like a cloud.
> And now my life ebbs away;
>> days of suffering grip me.
> Night pierces my bones;
>> my gnawing pains never rest.
> In his great power God becomes like clothing to me;
>> he binds me like the neck of his garment.
> He throws me into the mud,
>> and I am reduced to dust and ashes.
> I cry out to you, O God, but you do not answer;
>> I stand up, but you merely look at me. (Job 30:15-20)

Recently I visited on several occasions with a church friend who was suffering from advanced cancer of the lungs that had spread to the bones. The pain was sometimes excruciating and very difficult to bear. He felt God as being distant, but he courageously continued to exercise faith and prayed and cried out to God for mercy and help. The deepest and only prayer possible in such experiences of terrible pain may be simply to cry out, as he did: "O God, have mercy on me. Please help me!" All I could do was join in this same prayer on his behalf, pleading that God's mercy and presence would be with him.

Praying Through Chronic Pain

At times of persistent pain, you may also find the following prayer written by Richard Foster to be of particular help:

O Lord, my God, I do not ask for the pain to go away. I've prayed that prayer a thousand times over, and the pain remains with me. But I'm not angry about it. I'm not even disappointed anymore. I've come to terms with my pain.

No, my prayer is much more basic, much more simple. I ask, O God, for help in getting through this day. It's difficult because I've lost the ability to care.

God, what's hardest of all is that no one understands my experience of pain. If I had a broken leg, they could understand. But my pain is too hidden for them to understand. . . . And their doubts make me doubt myself, and when I doubt myself, it is hard to get through the day.

. . . Meaning has long since fled my life. What purpose is there in all this pain? Why am I here on this earth? What am I supposed to do with my life? These questions mock me.

I don't know who I am anymore, but whoever I am, O Lord, you know that I am thine. Amen.[9]

May the Lord keep you by his grace, and may he enable you to endure and pray through your chronic pain. And may those of us who do not suffer such pain learn, by God's grace, to be more understanding, empathic and patient with those who do.

Part Three
Conclusion

10

Putting It All Together

I N THIS CLOSING CHAPTER I WOULD LIKE TO HELP YOU PUT VARIOUS insights together in your attempts to live with or manage your chronic-pain condition in an effective way.

The earlier chapters of this book have given you a better understanding of pain as a complex experience that can be viewed as a problem, a puzzle—even a gift! They have also provided you with biblical perspectives on the power of God in pain and healing as well as the grace of God in pain and suffering. The major methods for pain control—medical and surgical methods, physical or sensory modulation methods, psychological and psychosocial methods, pain clinics and hospices, and spiritual methods—have been described for you so that you are now aware of the many strategies and options available for coping with pain and managing it more effectively. You can begin to use them as appropriate to your situation and your chronic pain in consultation with your medical doctor or specialist for your pain treatment.

Let's go back to the story of Bob, whom I described in chapter three. Bob's low-back pain had persisted for over a year despite his being on pain medications; it had become a *chronic* pain condition. Out of desperation he had decided to consult his orthopedic surgeon again concerning possible back surgery. Yet he still had some hesitation because of what he had read about the bad side effects and poor success rates of such surgery, especially when no clear-cut nerve or disc damage can be found. Let me tell you the rest of Bob's story.

The orthopedic surgeon described both the possible advantages and the risks, leaving the decision up to Bob. Bob almost decided to go ahead with the surgery. However, he made a last-minute decision to cancel it because his close friend Jon, who also had had low-back pain problems for a few years, told him that similar back surgery had not helped him at all.

Jon told Bob that several other pain-control methods had been more helpful to him as he learned to cope with his chronic low-back pain. The pain is still there, but Jon is suffering less from it. And the actual pain has also improved somewhat—it tends to be less intense when it occurs, and it has decreased in its frequency from daily to a couple of times a week.

Jon explained to Bob that most of the help he received had come from consulting a neurologist who specialized partly in pain treatment and, subsequently, from a clinical psychologist to whom the neurologist referred him. From them he had learned psychological and psychosocial methods as well as spiritual means for pain control. He eventually also consulted a pain clinic or pain treatment center at a well-known hospital, and the multidisciplinary team of pain doctors and other health-care professionals provided him with a few other pain-management strategies that helped him—without further surgery—to achieve even better pain control.

Bob was relieved to hear this account from his friend, and he proceeded immediately to set up an appointment with Jon's neurologist.

The neurologist examined Bob and, after consulting with Bob's orthopedic surgeon and going over the MRI and other medical findings, advised him to try several other methods of pain control before going for surgery. He referred Bob to a clinical psychologist who had some training and experience in psychological strategies for pain management, so that Bob could learn how to use such pain-control methods. The neurologist also started Bob on some TENS (transcutaneous electrical nerve stimulation) treatment in his lower-back area, and this brought him some pain relief.

Bob saw the clinical psychologist for several sessions. He learned to use the following psychological methods for pain control: relaxation techniques; calming self-talk; pleasant imagery; cognitive coping skills and distraction; cognitive therapy methods to change his negative, catastrophic, pessimistic thinking to more realistic, reasonable, hopeful or optimistic thinking regarding his pain; stress-inoculation training combining many of these mentioned so far; pacing and scheduling pleasurable activities.

The psychologist also helped him to include adequate rest and sleep, good nutrition and regular exercise (brisk walking three times a week for about thirty minutes each time) as part of his stress- and tension-management plan.

Finally, since they were both Christians and Bob wanted spiritual resources to be included in his therapy sessions, the psychologist also prayed with Bob for God's healing power and grace to touch him. Bob sought further prayer support and mutual encouragement from a church small group that had several members with chronic-pain problems. They met weekly to share, pray and encourage each other as well as study the Bible together. The psychologist had referred him to this small group after Bob expressed an interest in having more social and spiritual support in his life—a life which had been too busy and hectic up to that time for him to have much contact with church friends.

As Bob learned and used the various psychological and spiritual methods of pain control, he experienced even greater reduction of his low-back pain than what previous pain medications and even TENS had brought him. Although his pain did not go away completely, he was gradually able to control it more effectively.

His lifestyle had been modified: he spent more time now relaxing and resting, exercising regularly and socializing with good friends. His work schedule was still demanding, but he was careful not to overwork and not to lift heavy objects by himself.

His thinking and values had also changed. He was more reasonable and optimistic in how he looked at life; he valued much more his relationships with God and with people. Making money and having material things were no longer that important to him. He began to spend more time with God in prayer and in the Bible. He took periodic private retreats and really appreciated such times of solitude and personal renewal. He also had more frequent fellowship with his Christian friends and continued to attend the church small group for support. He therefore did not feel he needed to consult a pain clinic or treatment center. He had learned to manage his chronic pain effectively and live with pain successfully!

Not all chronic-pain patients or people suffering from low-back pain conditions end up like Bob. Some keep on struggling with intense and unrelenting pain, despite further surgery and all kinds of other pain treatment. Whatever your situation or experience may be, I encourage you to keep on using the pain-control methods you have learned through this book, in order to cope more effectively with pain in your life.

Steps for Coping with Pain
Sternbach has suggested the following steps for coping with chronic pain; you may find them helpful.

1. Accept the fact of having chronic pain.
2. Set specific goals for work, recreation or hobbies and social activities toward which you will work.
3. Let yourself get angry at the pain if it seems to be getting the best of you (rather than letting it get you down or depressed).
4. Take your analgesics or pain medications on a strict schedule,

and then taper them off.

5. Get in the best physical shape possible; then keep fit.
6. Learn how to relax, and practice relaxation regularly.
7. Keep yourself busy (but not too busy!).
8. Pace your activities.
9. Have your family and friends support only your healthy behavior, not your invalidism.
10. Be open and reasonable with your doctor.
11. Practice effective empathy with others having pain problems.
12. Remain hopeful.[1]

I would add another step from a Christian perspective: trust God through Jesus Christ, and exercise faith in him and his love and grace toward you, no matter what your circumstances might be or how bad your pain.

You can do this as you use the spiritual disciplines regularly in your life, applying spiritual means of pain control, including fellowship, prayer support and mutual encouragement with other Christians. The Holy Spirit will fill your heart with hope and God's love (Rom 5:5; 15:13) as you continue to pray and seek the Lord with all your heart. You will find him and know him ultimately to be a good, gracious and great God who also suffers with you, who has plans for you—plans not to harm you but to prosper you and give you hope and a future (Jer 29:11-13).

And ultimately that future includes an unending life in heaven, where God will wipe every tear from your eyes, where you shall no more experience any pain, or mourning, or crying, or death, for the old order of things will have passed away! (Rev 21:4).

God's Promised Presence

Meanwhile, even on earth, in this fallen and trouble-filled life with its ups and downs, joys and tribulations, he has promised to be with you (Mt 28:20; Heb 13:5-6) and to give you his peace (Jn 16:33). He has promised to work in *all* things for the good of those who love him and have been called according to his purpose (Rom 8:28). So, even through trials, afflictions and pain, we can grow in genuine, deep faith and fidelity (see 1 Pet 1:6-7) and develop perseverance, maturity and Christlike character (see Jas 1:2-4).

God is still, and always will be, up to some good, not no good! And nothing, nothing at all, not even unrelenting chronic pain, can separate us from his love for us that is in Christ Jesus our Lord (Rom 8:31-39).

Yet Philip Yancey has pointed out that we often long for shortcuts to spiritual growth and maturity in faith, much like the schoolboys who want to quickly get the answers to their math problems by looking in the back of the book instead of working them through. Yancey writes:

> We yearn for shortcuts. But shortcuts usually lead away from growth, not toward it. Apply the principle directly to Job: what was the final result of the testing he went through? As Rabbi Abraham Heschel observed, "Faith like Job's cannot be shaken because it is the result of having been shaken."[2]

It may be helpful for all of us to remember what God has truly promised us regarding life on earth—a life that is often so difficult. In the words of Annie Johnson Flint:

God hath not promised skies always blue
Flower strewn pathways all our lives thru
God hath not promised sun without rain
Joy without sorrow, peace without pain.

God hath not promised we shall not know
Toil and temptation, trouble and woe
He hath not told us we shall not bear
Many a burden, many a care.

But God hath promised strength for the day

Rest for the labor, light for the way
Grace for the trials, help from above
Unfailing sympathy, undying love.[3]

We do not have all the answers we would like to have to life's per-
plexing, complex questions—of which the problem or puzzle of pain
remains one of the most difficult and challenging. Melzack and Wall
have concluded:

> Ultimately, the greatest challenge of pain continues to be the pa-
> tient who has received every known treatment yet continues to
> suffer. No matter how splendid the progress in recent years in pain
> research and treatment, there are still large numbers of people
> who fail to respond to the best efforts of all the best therapists.
> These people—with excruciating cancer, post-herpetic neuralgia,
> low back pain—are the true measure of our knowledge and capa-
> bility. Until we have learned to control this suffering the challenge
> of pain is as great as ever.[4]

In the context of such a continuing challenge of pain, Drs. Oates and
Oates offer us the following realistic benediction or closing blessing:
"May you heal sometimes, remedy often, and comfort always in the
name of our Lord Jesus Christ."[5]

As you learn to put it all together in managing chronic pain, remember that the Christian perspective gives you the deepest love and
greatest hope through Jesus Christ, our Lord and Savior. Underneath
you and your struggles with chronic pain and suffering will always be
God's everlasting arms of love (Deut 33:27; compare Rom 8:35-39). His
word to you is this:

> The LORD your God is with you, he is mighty to save. He will take
> great delight in you, he will quiet you with his love, he will rejoice
> over you with singing! (Zeph 3:17)

And may your response and mine become more and more like Ha-
bakkuk's:

> Though the fig tree does not bud

   and there are no grapes on the vines,
though the olive crop fails
   and the fields produce no food,
though there are no sheep in the pen
   and no cattle in the stalls,
yet I will rejoice in the LORD,
   I will be joyful in God my Savior.
The Sovereign LORD is my strength;
   he makes my feet like the feet of a deer,
   he enables me to go on the heights. (Hab 3:17-19)

Notes

Chapter 1: Pain: Problem, Puzzle or Gift?

[1]Ronald Melzack and Patrick D. Wall, *The Challenge of Pain* (New York: Basic Books, 1983), p. 9.

[2]International Association for the Study of Pain, Subcommittee on Taxonomy, "Pain Terms: A List with Definitions and Notes on Its Usage," *Pain* 6 (1979): 249-52.

[3]John J. Bonica, foreword to *Mastering Pain: A Twelve-Step Program for Coping with Chronic Pain* by Richard A. Sternbach (New York: Putnam, 1987), p. 11.

[4]Wayne E. Oates and Charles E. Oates, *People in Pain: Guidelines for Pastoral Care* (Philadelphia: Westminster Press, 1985).

[5]Thomas W. Miller, "Concluding Thoughts on Chronic Pain," in *Chronic Pain*, vol. 2, ed. Thomas W. Miller (Madison, Conn.: International Universities Press, 1990), p. 840.

[6]Sternbach, *Mastering Pain*, p. 15.

[7]Richard W. Hanson and Kenneth E. Gerber, *Coping with Chronic Pain: A Guide to Patient Self-Management* (New York: Guilford Press, 1990), pp. 2-3. Also see M. Osterweis, A. Kleinman and D. Mechanic, eds., *Pain and Disability: Clinical, Behavioral and Public Policy Perspectives* (Washington, D.C.: National Academy Press, 1987).

[8]H. Taylor and N. Curran, *The Nuprin Pain Report* (New York: Louis Harris & Associates, 1985). Also see Sternbach, *Mastering Pain*, pp. 14-15.

[9]Melzack and Wall, *Challenge of Pain*, pp. 15-26.

[10]Paul Brand and Philip Yancey, *Pain: The Gift Nobody Wants* (Grand Rapids, Mich.: Zondervan, 1993).

Chapter 2: Understanding Pain
[1]H. K. Beecher, *Measurement of Subjective Responses* (New York: Oxford University Press, 1959).
[2]Ronald Melzack, "Pain: Past, Present and Future," *Canadian Journal of Experimental Psychology* 47 (1993): 615-29. Also see Melzack and Wall, *Challenge of Pain.*
[3]Ronald Melzack and Patrick D. Wall, "Pain Mechanisms: A New Theory," *Science* 150 (1965): 971-79. Also see Melzack, "Pain: Past, Present and Future"; Melzack and Wall, *Challenge of Pain.*
[4]Melzack, "Pain: Past, Present and Future." Also see Ronald Melzack, "Phantom Limbs, the Self and the Brain (The D.O. Hebb Memorial Lecture)," *Canadian Psychology* 30 (1989): 1-14.
[5]Sternbach, *Mastering Pain,* p. 36.
[6]Ibid., pp. 38-39.
[7]See Siang-Yang Tan, "Pain," in *Baker Encyclopedia of Psychology,* ed. David G. Benner (Grand Rapids, Mich.: Baker Book House, 1985), pp. 785-86. Also see David Morris, *The Culture of Pain* (Berkeley: University of California Press, 1991).
[8]Ellen Catalano, *The Chronic Pain Control Workbook* (Oakland, Calif.: New Harbinger Publications, 1987).
[9]See Tan, "Pain," and Siang-Yang Tan, "Cognitive and Cognitive-Behavioral Methods for Pain Control: A Selective Review," *Pain* 12 (1982): 201-28.
[10]Sternbach, *Mastering Pain,* p. 31.
[11]D. C. Turk, D. Meichenbaum and M. Genest, *Pain and Behavioral Medicine: A Cognitive-Behavioral Perspective* (New York: Guilford, 1983).
[12]See Dennis C. Turk and Ronald Melzack, eds., *Handbook of Pain Assessment* (New York: Guilford, 1992).
[13]Ronald Melzack, "The McGill Pain Questionnaire: Major Properties and Scoring Methods," *Pain* 1 (1975): 277-99. Also see Ronald Melzack, "The Short-Form McGill Pain Questionnaire," *Pain* 30 (1987): 191-97.

Chapter 3: Medical & Surgical Methods for Pain Control
[1]Hanson and Gerber, *Coping with Chronic Pain,* pp. 3-4.
[2]Ibid., p. 5.
[3]Melzack and Wall, *Challenge of Pain,* p. 269.
[4]Eric J. Cassel, "Introduction: The Nature of Suffering and the Goals of Medicine," in *Chronic Pain,* vol. 1, ed. Thomas W. Miller (Madison, Conn.: International Universities Press, 1990), pp. xxiv-xxv.
[5]Ibid., p. xxii.
[6]See Ronald Melzack and Patrick Wall, *The Challenge of Pain,* rev. ed. (Harmondsworth, Middlesex, England: Penguin Books, 1988), pp. 197-213.
[7]See Sternbach, *Mastering Pain,* pp. 69-73.
[8]See Charles B. Stacy, Andrew S. Kaplan and Gray Williams Jr., *The Fight Against Pain* (Yonkers, N. Y.: Consumer Reports Books, 1992), pp. 168-201.

[9]See Frank Minirth, *The Headache Book* (Nashville, Tenn.: Nelson, 1994), p. 77.
[10]See Sternbach, *Mastering Pain*, pp. 145-61.
[11]Ibid., pp. 60-64.
[12]Melzack and Wall, *Challenge of Pain*, pp. 285-98.

Chapter 4: Sensory Modulation & Other Physical Methods for Pain Control
[1]See Melzack and Wall, *Challenge of Pain*, pp. 299-331.
[2]Sternbach, *Mastering Pain*, p. 68.
[3]Catalano, *Chronic Pain Control Workbook*, p. 19.
[4]Ibid., pp. 18-19.
[5]Stacy, Kaplan and Williams, *The Fight Against Pain*, p. 152.
[6]See Melzack and Wall, *Challenge of Pain*, pp. 319-31.
[7]See Catalano, *Chronic Pain Control Workbook*, pp. 25-40.
[8]Bryant A. Stamford and Porter Shimer, *Fitness Without Exercise* (New York: Warner Books, 1990).
[9]David Zemach-Bersin, Kaethe Zemach-Bersin and Mark Reese, *Relaxercise* (San Francisco: Harper & Row, 1990).
[10]Stamford and Shimer, *Fitness Without Exercise*, pp. 125-87.
[11]Margaret A. Caudill, *Managing Pain Before It Manages You* (New York: Guilford, 1995), pp. 90-91.
[12]See Archibald D. Hart, *Adrenaline and Stress*, rev. ed. (Dallas: Word, 1995).

Chapter 5: Psychological & Psychosocial Methods for Pain Control
[1]See Tan, "Cognitive and Cognitive-Behavioral Methods for Pain Control"; Turk, Meichenbaum and Genest, *Pain and Behavioral Medicine*. Also see Catalano, *Chronic Pain Control Workbook;* Caudill, *Managing Pain;* Robert J. Gatchel and Dennis C. Turk, eds., *Psychological Approaches to Pain Management: A Practitioner's Handbook* (New York: Guilford, 1996); Hanson and Gerber, *Coping with Chronic Pain;* Melzack and Wall, *Challenge of Pain*, rev. ed.; Sternbach, *Mastering Pain*.
[2]Caudill, *Managing Pain*, p. 49.
[3]See Turk, Meichenbaum and Genest, *Pain and Behavioral Medicine*.
[4]Herbert Benson, *The Relaxation Response* (New York: William Morrow, 1975).
[5]Tan, "Cognitive and Cognitive-Behavioral Methods for Pain Control," p. 206.
[6]Jon Kabat-Zinn, *Full Catastrophe Living: Using the Wisdom of Your Body and Mind to Face Stress, Pain and Illness* (New York: Delta, 1990), pp. 283-318.
[7]See William Backus and Marie Chapian, *Telling Yourself the Truth* (Minneapolis, Minn.: Bethany, 1980); William Backus, *Telling the Truth to Troubled People* (Minneapolis, Minn.: Bethany, 1985); Mark McMinn, *Cognitive Therapy Techniques in Christian Counseling* (Dallas: Word, 1991); Rebecca Propst, *Psychotherapy in a Religious Framework: Spirituality in the Emotional Healing Process* (New York: Human Sciences Press, 1988); David Stoop, *Self-Talk: Key to Personal Growth*, 2d ed. (Grand Rapids, Mich.: Revell, 1996); Chris Thurman, *The Lies We Believe* (Nashville, Tenn.: Nelson, 1989); H. Nor-

man Wright, *Self-Talk, Imagery and Prayer in Counseling* (Waco, Tex.: Word, 1986). Also see Siang-Yang Tan, "Cognitive-Behavior Therapy: A Biblical Approach and Critique," *Journal of Psychology and Theology* 15 (1987): 103-12; Siang-Yang Tan and John Ortberg Jr., *Understanding Depression* (Grand Rapids, Mich.: Baker Book House, 1995); and Siang-Yang Tan and John Ortberg Jr., *Coping with Depression* (Grand Rapids, Mich.: Baker Book House, 1995).

[8]David Burns, *Feeling Good* (New York: Signet, 1980). Also see Tan and Ortberg, *Coping with Depression* (chapter 6).

[9]Thurman, *Lies We Believe.*

[10]Donald Meichenbaum, *Stress Inoculation Training* (New York: Pergamon Press, 1985). Also see Donald Meichenbaum, "Stress Inoculation Training: A 20-Year Update," in Paul M. Lehrer and Robert L. Woolfolk, eds., *Principles and Practice of Stress Management,* 2nd ed. (New York: Guilford Press, 1993), pp. 373-406.

[11]Melzack and Wall, *Challenge of Pain,* rev. ed., p. 260.

[12]Ibid., pp. 246-47.

[13]Ibid., pp. 247-49.

[14]Jean Holroyd, "Hypnosis Treatment of Clinical Pain: Understanding Why Hypnosis Is Useful," *International Journal of Clinical and Experimental Hypnosis* 44 (1996): 33-51.

[15]Melzack and Wall, *The Challenge of Pain,* rev. ed., pp. 252-56. Also see William E. Fordyce, *Behavioral Methods for Chronic Pain and Illness* (St. Louis, Mo.: C. V. Mosby, 1976).

[16]Sternbach, *Mastering Pain,* pp. 121-26.

[17]Melzack and Wall, *Challenge of Pain,* rev. ed., pp. 257-58.

[18]Ibid., p. 261.

[19]Francis J. Keefe, Julie Dunsmore and Rachel Burnett, "Behavioral and Cognitive-Behavioral Approaches to Chronic Pain: Recent Advances and Future Directions," *Journal of Consulting and Clinical Psychology* 60 (1992): 528-36.

Chapter 6: Pain Clinics & Hospices

[1]Melzack and Wall, *Challenge of Pain,* pp. 356-77.

[2]Sternbach, *Mastering Pain,* appendix A, pp. 218-23.

[3]Francis J. Keefe, Karen M. Gil and Sandra C. Rose, "Behavioral Approaches in the Multidisciplinary Management of Chronic Pain: Programs and Issues," *Clinical Psychology Review* 6 (1986): 87-113.

[4]J. J. Bonica, "Cancer Pain," in *Pain,* ed. J. J. Bonica (New York: Raven Press, 1980), pp. 335-62.

Chapter 7: Pain & Healing: The Power of God

[1]For example, see Colin Brown, *That You May Believe: Miracles and Faith, Then and Now* (Grand Rapids, Mich.: Eerdmans, 1985); Jack Deere, *Surprised by the Power of the Spirit* (Grand Rapids, Mich.: Zondervan, 1993); Rex Gardner, *Healing Miracles: A Doctor Investigates* (London: Darton, Longman & Todd, 1986); Michael Harper, *The Healings of Jesus* (Downers Grove, Ill.: InterVarsity Press, 1986); Lewis B. Smedes, ed., *Ministry*

and the Miraculous: A Case Study at Fuller Theological Seminary (Pasadena, Calif.: Fuller Theological Seminary, 1987); C. Peter Wagner, *How to Have a Healing Ministry in Any Church* (Ventura, Calif.: Regal, 1988); John Wimber with Kevin Springer, *Power Healing* (San Francisco: Harper & Row, 1987).

[2]See Wimber with Springer, *Power Healing*, pp. xviii-xix, 129.

[3]William Barclay, *The Daily Study Bible: The Gospel of Mark*, rev. ed. (Edinburgh: Saint Andrew Press, 1975), p. 40.

[4]C. Peter Wagner, *Your Spiritual Gifts Can Help Your Church Grow*, rev. ed. (Ventura, Calif.: Regal, 1994), p. 210.

[5]See Wimber with Springer, *Power Healing*, pp. 140-42.

[6]Ibid., pp. 147-52.

[7]Ibid., pp. 145-46.

[8]Michael E. McCullough, "Prayer and Health: Conceptual Issues, Research Review and Research Agenda," *Journal of Psychology and Theology* 23 (1995): 15-29. Also see J. A. Turner and S. Clancy, "Strategies for Coping with Chronic Low Back Pain: Relationship to Pain and Disability," *Pain* 24 (1986): 355-64.

Chapter 8: Spiritual Means of Pain Control

[1]Richard J. Foster, *Prayer: Finding the Heart's True Home* (San Francisco: HarperCollins, 1992), pp. 1-2.

[2]Richard J. Foster, in *RENOVARÉ Perspective* (vol. 1, no. 2), a publication of RENOVARÉ, an organization committed to spiritual renewal, which he heads. For further information on RENOVARÉ and how to receive *RENOVARÉ Perspective* several times a year, write to RENOVARÉ, 8 Inverness Drive East, Suite 102, Englewood, CO 80112-5609, call (303) 792-0152 or fax (303) 792-0146.

[3]Brand and Yancey, *Pain: The Gift Nobody Wants*, pp. 286-87.

[4]James Dobson, *When God Doesn't Make Sense* (Wheaton, Ill.: Tyndale, 1993).

[5]Richard J. Foster, *Celebration of Discipline*, rev. ed. (San Francisco: Harper & Row, 1988).

[6]David Ray, *The Art of Christian Meditation* (Wheaton, Ill.: Tyndale, 1977), pp. 53-56.

[7]Jay E. Adams, *Ready to Restore: The Layman's Guide to Christian Counseling* (Grand Rapids, Mich.: Baker Book House, 1981), pp. 64-65.

[8]William L. Conwill, "Chronic Pain Conceptualization and Religious Interpretation," *Journal of Religion and Health* 25 (1986): 24-50.

[9]Avie J. Rainwater III, "Understanding the Suffering of Chronic Pain," *Journal of Psychology and Christianity* 14 (1995): 170-77.

[10]Ellie T. Sturgis, "The Relationship Between a Personal Theology and Chronic Pain," in *Behavior Therapy and Religion: Integrating Spiritual and Behavioral Approaches to Change*, ed. William R. Miller and John E. Martin (Newbury Park, Calif.: SAGE, 1988), pp. 111-23. Also see Oates and Oates, *People in Pain*.

Chapter 9: Pain & Suffering: The Grace of God

[1]Philip Yancey, *Where Is God When It Hurts?* rev. ed. (Grand Rapids, Mich.: Zondervan,

1990).

[2]Philip Yancey, *Disappointment with God: Three Questions No One Asks Aloud* (Grand Rapids, Mich.: Zondervan, 1988).

[3]Glandion Carney and William Long, *Trusting God Again* (Downers Grove, Ill.: Inter-Varsity Press, 1995), p. 64.

[4]Yancey, *Where Is God When It Hurts?* p. 234.

[5]Ibid., pp. 256-57.

[6]Sturgis, "Relationship Between a Personal Theology and Chronic Pain," p. 117.

[7]Ibid., pp. 117-18.

[8]Yancey, *Disappointment with God,* p. 244.

[9]Richard J. Foster, *Prayers from the Heart* (San Francisco: HarperCollins, 1994), p. 12.

Chapter 10: Putting It All Together

[1]Sternbach, *Mastering Pain,* pp. 211-17.

[2]Yancey, *Disappointment with God,* p. 208.

[3]First two stanzas and chorus taken from "God Hath Not Promised," hymn 362, written by Annie Johnson Flint and published without copyright in *Hymns for God's People* (Glendale, Calif.: Hymns for God's People, 1984).

[4]Melzack and Wall, *Challenge of Pain,* p. 403.

[5]Oates and Oates, *People in Pain,* p. 134.